THE ANTIOXIDANT COOKBOOK

OTHER BOOKS BY MICHAEL WEINER, Ph.D.

Herbs that Heal
Maximum Immunity
Nutrition Against Aging
The Skeptical Nutritionist
Earth Medicine: Earth Foods
The Complete Book of Homeopathy
Secrets of Fijian Medicine
Weiner's Herbal
Healing Children Naturally
The Herbal Bible
Man's Useful Plants
Plant-A-Tree: A Guide to Regreening America
Reducing the Risk of Alzheimer's Disease
Hi-Fiber Counter
Herbs & Immunity

THE ANTIOXIDANT COOKBOOK

By
Michael A. Weiner, Ph.D.
and
Terri Chantrelle

A
QUANTUM
BOOK

THE ANTIOXIDANT COOKBOOK

Printed in the United States of America

PUBLISHER:
Quantum Books
Six Knoll Lane
Mill Valley, CA 94941 USA

EDITOR:
Janet Weiner

ILLUSTRATIONS:
Terry Chantrelle

TYPESETTING:
Wordsworth, San Geronimo, CA

Library of Congress Cataloging in Publication Data:
Card Number 95-078906
Weiner, Michael A., & Chantrelle, Terri
ISBN 0-912845-13-9
The Antioxidant Cookbook
280 pages, 150 illustrations
Includes References & Index
1. COOKBOOK - ANTI-AGING RECIPES
2. HEALTH & FITNESS - COOKBOOK
3. DIET & LONGEVITY
4. HEART HEALTH

We want to thank our friends & family
for the encouragement given during
the gestation of this book.

For
Bette & Charles,
from Terri.

For
Becky, Laura, Larry & Robina
from Janet.

For
Rae & Benny
from Michael

TABLE OF CONTENTS

INTRODUCTION

FROM THE EDITOR

This cookbook was born of the collaborative creative talents of two wonderful people, who believe that people need to eat delicious, easy to prepare meals that are also guaranteed to supply high antioxidant superfood value. In so doing, careful attention has been paid to concurrently insure low calorie, low fat, low cholesterol, low salt, sugar free, high potency superfoods.

The primary keynote of all the recipes contained in the following pages are that they are *simple to prepare*. All the ingredients are readily available in local markets, and the dishes themselves require very little advance planning or preparation time. Cooking times are quick. The focus is on simple, antioxidant-rich ingredients, for all the recipes.

Dr. Michael Weiner received his Ph.D. in Nutritional Ethno-Medicine from the University of California at Berkeley. He also holds an M.A. degree in Medical Anthropology and an M.S. degree in Ethnobotany. Dr. Weiner's many books include: *Maximum Immunity, Nutrition Against Aging, Herbs that Heal, The Complete Book of Homeopathy, Healing Children Naturally, The Herbal Bible*, and *The Way of the Skeptical Nutritionist*. In all of these books, Dr. Weiner has sought to apply his keen scientific training to elucidate the ethnic wisdom of the world's diverse cultures, particularly, why do peoples from various traditional cultures eat certain foods? What can we learn from them? Dr. Weiner is a master cook and has spent twenty-five years developing and fine-tuning the special methods you will learn of in this volume.

After Dr. Weiner developed the concept for this book, he searched for years to find the right coauthor. Happily, Terri Chantrelle, a New York born, long-time San Francisco resident, made Dr. Weiner's acquaintance. Terri comes from a multi-ethnic background, as varied as the spices and ingredients she uses in her recipes. She has done design work and is an accomplished illustrator as well as a published cartoonist. Terri is a much sought after hotel and restaurant chef in San Francisco.

Dr. Weiner and Terri proceeded to cook up a storm together! The results are in and the scorecards rates them A+! Dr. Weiner's scientific background in nutrition guarantees these recipes are designed to significantly reduce your risk of heart disease, cancer, diabetes, and arthritis. Further added benefits of this antioxidant diet are:

- fortification of the brain and nervous system against memory disability;
- the promotion of active weight loss and athletic vigor;
- the maintenance of healthy skin, nails, and lustrous hair;
- enhanced sensory competence, particularly vision enhancement.

Yet, with Dr. Weiner's secret strategy and Terri's magic touch—these recipes are delicious! Your family and friends will be amazed that food that tastes this *great* is so good for them!

Superfoods!

A nutritionists secret strategy for delicious and healthy eating!

We have already described how these recipes are low calories, low fat, low cholesterol, low salt, sugar-free, high potency superfoods to boost your antioxidant quotient.

Now let's explain why antioxidant rich foods are so important. You have all heard the term—

Antioxidant

But — Just what does that mean?
And — Why is it important?

Antioxidant. A powerful word. Simply explained, the body's cells, during the normal metabolic process—called oxidation—of burning fuel (food) to produce energy for all the organs and systems, produces *free radicals*. These *free radicals* are a normal byproduct of the oxidation process. In today's world, due to our extraordinary exposure to pollution, environmental toxins, carbon monoxide, over-exposure to the sun's rays, and other threatening elements, our production of *free radicals* has increased beyond what our cells were originally designed to handle. This excessive amount of free radical elements in our bodies leads to the maiming and destruction of our cells' membranes and genetic material. This can lead to premature aging, neurological disorders, cancer, cataracts, other diseases, and death before our time. So, the key is to diminish free radical production, or destroy the free radicals!

Leave a cut piece of apple on your kitchen counter for a few hours and observe the changes. The browning of the fruit, the puckering of the skin. This shows all too clearly how free radicals can ravage our interior and exterior beings. Or, imagine a rusty piece of metal. Same concept. Over-oxidation.

> Antioxidants are substances that help prevent the production of free radicals. It's that simple. This book takes the worry out of recipe planning. When you make one of these meals, you will clearly see—printed adjacent to the menu—exactly which antioxidants you are getting in that meal.

We now know many of the antioxidants. In order of importance, they are: vitamin A, vitamin C, vitamin E, Beta and Alpha Carotene (also known as the carotenoids), Lycopene, and Lutein. It has been demonstrated conclusively in scientific studies that the addition of antioxidant nutrients to the human diet will assist with the prevention of disease and premature aging.

ANTIOXIDANT VITAMINS

VITAMIN A

Vitamin A, or retinol, has long been known to promote *nonspecific* resistance to a wide variety of pathogens. This is partly due to its involvement in the production of mucopolysaccharide, a component of the *mucous membranes*. An early sign of vitamin A deficiency is damage to the linings of the respiratory, digestive, and urogenital tracts. By helping to preserve the integrity of skin and mucous membranes, vitamin A helps to maintain the protective barriers against infectious organisms entering the body. Vitamin A is also needed for the production of bacteria-fighting lysozymes in tears, saliva, and sweat.

Recent research has shown that vitamin A also has a powerful effect on *specific* immune system functions, stimulating both cell-mediated and humoral immunity. Studies of animals with vitamin A deficiency have shown atrophy of thymus and lymphoid tissue, decrease in total number of T and B cells, and depression of T cell response to mitogens and antibody response to infectious agents, including bacteria, viruses, and fungi. Vitamin A deficiency increases susceptibility to viral, bacterial, and protozoal infections and makes these problems worse and more often fatal. Other immune system changes associated with vitamin A deficiency include decreased T to B cell ratio, T and B cell proliferative response, spleen cell response, delayed skin sensitivity, monocyte (a kind of white cell) function, and inflammatory response.

Most studies of the immunological effects of vitamin A have employed laboratory animals with a deficiency of the vitamin. In contrast, a study by Cohen et al. describes the use of megadoses of vitamin A in humans who had had minor surgery. As a result of surgery, people often experience a suppression of immune function for weeks, with a decrease in cell-mediated immunity and in macrophage and neutrophil function. This immunosuppression may be a result of the stress related to surgery and/or an effect of anesthesia.

In the Cohen study, patients scheduled for extensive surgery were divided into two groups; one was given large daily doses of vitamin A, and the other served as a control. Blood samples were collected one day before surgery, one day after surgery, and seven days after surgery. The vitamin A treated group showed increased T cell activity seven days after surgery, while the control group showed the usual immunosuppression. Thus vitamin A was shown to be capable of blocking the suppression of immune function that is often associated with surgery.

The patients in this study received very large doses, 300,000 to 450,000 IU, of vitamin A daily, for one week after surgery. It is noteworthy that there were no signs of toxicity from these megadoses. When taken in excessive amounts, vitamin A produces a characteristic toxicity pattern of headache, vomiting, vertigo, blurred vision, liver damage, and sometimes yellowing of the skin. In fact, vitamin A toxicity is the most common form of any vitamin toxicity, largely because vitamin A is oil soluble. Whereas water-soluble vitamins are constantly being flushed out of the system, vitamin A can accumulate in the body's fat cells, building up to a level where symptoms appear. Because of the possibility of overdose, many people have shied away from vitamin A, even though the toxicity is easily corrected by reducing the vitamin's intake. The absence of toxic symptoms in the above study should help to reassure you of the safety of this important protective vitamin.

Vitamin A appears to be one of the most important protective nutrients against cancer. In studies using animals or human blood samples, various forms of vitamin A seemed to reduce the conversion of altered cells into cancerous cells and to protect against tumors induced by chemical carcinogens. More recently a study in the Philippines found that high weekly doses of vitamin A and vitamin A precursor helped protect chewers of betel nut and tobacco leaf from chromosome breaks and oral cancer. Users of these substances have a high rate of oral cancer. Vitamin A also appears to be generally protective against the immune-suppressing effects of stress.

Green and yellow fruits and vegetables are an important source of vitamin A (in decreasing order, beginning with those highest in vitamin A content: carrots, sweet potatoes, spinach, cantaloupe, apricots, broccoli, peaches, cherries, tomatoes, and asparagus). Milk and milk products, beef liver, and fish liver oil are other sources of this important protective vitamin.

VITAMIN C (ASCORBIC ACID)

When Nobel laureate Linus Pauling first announced that high doses of vitamin C helped to prevent or lessen the severity of viral diseases such as the common cold and influenza, the public rushed to stock up on this nutrient. Researchers, seeking to verify or disprove Pauling's claims, generally did not use the high doses recommended by Pauling; but even at doses of less than one gram a day, most workers found that vitamin C reduced the severity of viral upper respiratory illnesses. Orthomolecular practitioners, using doses of at least 10 grams of vitamin C a day, report even greater benefits in reducing the symptoms of bacterial and viral diseases. Nor is it just minor illnesses such as the common cold and flu that are influenced by vitamin C. According to case studies by Dr. Robert Cathcart, this vitamin, when taken in a balanced nutritional program, also speeds recovery from mononucleosis and viral pneumonia.

Surprisingly, vitamin C deficiency has no apparent effect on most parts of the immune system, including the thymus and other lymphoid tissues, the T and B cells, and the antibodies. The beneficial immunological effects of vitamin C seem to be due to its enhancement of phagocytic functions—specifically, its stimulation of the motility of macrophages and neutrophils. This very specific effect of vitamin C has been confirmed by a study involving subjects with Chédiak-Higashi syndrome, a condition in which the neutrophils have low motility. Vitamin C was able to stimulate neutrophil motility in these people at the relatively low dose of 200 milligrams a day. To a much more limited extent, vitamin C may also have an influence on the ability of phagocytes to kill bacteria and fungi.

It remains a mystery how vitamin C improves our immunity against viruses. The vitamin appears to have no direct antiviral effect when examined outside the body. Recent studies suggest that vitamin C may stimulate T and B cell transformation, which means the vitamin does have an effect on cell-mediated immunity and may help explain it antiviral properties. If vitamin C enhances T cell function, it may also promote the release of interferons, which attack viruses.

One of the most exciting areas of vitamin C research is its therapeutic use in treating cancers. Drs. Linus Pauling and Ewan Cameron, a Scottish cancer surgeon, have reported that a dose of 10 grams a day is beneficial in some cancer cases, while Robert F. Cathcart III, M.D., Los Altos, California, uses much higher doses. According to Dr. Cathcart, the more serious the illness, the more vitamin C we need. Proper dose is determined by giving increasing amounts of ascorbic acid up to the point where diarrhea occurs, and then reducing the dosage by 10 percent. The dosage at which the bowel symptoms are produced is known as the *bowel tolerance level*. In the case of cancer, proper dosage can be as high as 100 grams a day.

How does vitamin C fight cancer? Since macrophages are believed to play a critical role in fighting tumors, the macrophage-stimulating properties of vitamin C would help to explain its beneficial effects. Moreover, the vitamin's stimulation of T cell transformation would help increase the antibody response to the tumor and stimulate the production of T killer cells, which destroy cancer cells.

Aspirin has an anti-vitamin C effect, promoting the loss of vitamin C through the urine and also decreasing uptake of the vitamin by white blood cells. Taking aspirin also seems to increase the danger of a spreading viral infection, as has been observed in Reye's syndrome in children. For these reasons, you may want to think twice before taking aspirin along with vitamin C for your cold or flu.

In its role as an antioxidant and free radical scavenger, vitamin C further helps to fight cancer by preventing the formation of carcinogens in the body. For example, ascorbic acid inhibits the formation of nitrosamines by reacting with nitrite before the nitrite can combine with amines in the diet to form the highly carcinogenic nitrosamines. As an antioxidant, vitamin C protects against lipid peroxidation, preventing the formation of dangerous free radicals. It has a synergistic effect when taken with other antioxidants: the more vitamin C you take, the less vitamin E you need.

In helping to combat the adverse effects of stress, vitamin C helps to counteract the immunosuppressive effects of corticosteroids, yet at the same time assists in the anti-inflammatory function of the steroids.

Besides its specific effects on immune functioning, ascorbic acid is also critical to bone and tooth formation, collagen production, and other forms of tissue integrity. Thus this vitamin is essential in maintaining your body's external defenses against infection.

Dietary sources of vitamin C, beginning with those highest in vitamin C concentration are: green peppers, broccoli, brussels sprouts, cauliflower, strawberries, spinach, oranges, cabbage, grapefruit, cantaloupe, and papaya. Because your body may require much higher amounts of vitamin C than can be obtained from food alone, Dr. Pauling and many other proponents of this amazing vitamin advocate daily consumption of vitamin C supplement as a protective measure.

VITAMIN E

Hailed in recent years as a "miracle vitamin," vitamin E is best known for its antioxidant properties. It is much less recognized for its ability to stimulate the immune system and to protect against infection.

Adding extra vitamin E to the diet of animals has ben shown to significantly enhance their ability to produce antibodies in response to pathogen exposure. Giving vitamin E in conjunction with selenium enhances the immune-boosting effects even further.

Most research on nutrients investigates the effects of deficiencies. Vitamin E deficiency has been shown to result in decreased lymphatic organ size, T and B cell proliferation, white blood cell function, inflammatory response, and host resistance to infection. In the case of vitamin E, much more work has been done on the effects of larger than normal doses, rather than on artificially created deficiencies. Elevated levels of vitamin E, in addition to producing enhanced antibody response, have been observed to improve white cell bactericidal activity, phagocytosis, and host resistance. Dietary supplements of vitamin E enhanced T helper cell activity in mice and vitamin E supplements may also help to reduce the immunosuppressive effects of corticosteroids.

Vitamin E is a powerful antioxidant that prevents the formation of free radicals and protects cell membranes against lipid peroxidation. These antioxidant and free radical scavenging properties help to protect against cancer in a variety of ways. For example, vitamin E helps to block the formation of carcinogenic nitrosamines out of nitrites in foods. In animal studies, vitamin E, added to food or applied to the skin, decreased the severity and number of tumors produced by carcinogenic substances.

In the process of killing bacteria, *macrophages produce free radicals*. High doses of vitamin E, as well as the antioxidant mineral selenium, help to protect macrophages from damage by these bactericidal free radicals.

The antioxidant properties of vitamin E also protect the lungs from air pollution damage.

Among its other important properties, vitamin E protects against dangerous blood clots and affects blood cholesterol levels, blood flow to the heart, strength of capillary walls, and muscle and nerve maintenance. It protects against stress in general, and some forms of vitamin E seem to increase fertility in laboratory animals.

Vitamin E is found in dark green vegetables, eggs, liver and other organ meats, wheat germ, vegetable oils, oatmeal, peanuts, and tomatoes.

PLANTS CONTAINING ANTIOXIDANTS

Additionally, naturally occurring oxidants are to be found in abundance in the plant kingdom in the following:

Acerola	Curry powder	Onion, green	Sage
Algae	Dill	Onion, red bermuda	Sarsaparilla
Apple cider	Eggplant	Onion, white	Sassafras
Apples	Eggplant, Japanese	Onion, yellow	Scallions
Apricots	Garlic	Orange, whole	Seaweeds
Asparagus	Ginger	Orange, juice	Sesame seeds
Bay leaf	Grapes	Orange, peel	Shallots
Bean sprouts	Guava	Oregano	Soy sauce
Beans, white	Honey	Papaya	Spearmint
Beans, pinto	Leeks	Paprika	Spinach
Beans, green	Lemon, whole	Parsley	Squash, yellow
Beans, kidney	Lemon, juice	Parsley, Italian	Tabasco sauce
Beans, black	Lemon, peel	Peaches	Tangelos
Berries	Lettuce, butter	Peanut butter	Tangerines
Broccoli	Lettuce, iceberg	Peas, green	Tarragon
Cabbage	Lettuce, romaine	Peas, snow	Thyme
Cantaloupe	Lettuce, wild	Pepper, black	Tomatoes, fresh
Carrots	Licorice	Pepper, cayenne	Tomatoes, sundried
Cashews	Lime	Pepper, white	Turmeric
Cauliflower	Mandarin oranges	Pepper, green bell	Vanilla
Celery	Mango	Pepper, red bell	Vinegar, apple cider
Cheese, cheddar	Mayonnaise	Pepper, yellow bell	Vinegar, red
Cheese, parmesan	Milk, lo-fat	Peppermint	Vinegar, rice
Cheese, ricotta	Milk thistle	Pine nuts	Vinegar, white
Cherries	Mint	Plum	Vinegar, red wine
Chili oil	Mushrooms, reishi	Pomegranate	Vinegar, white wine
Chili paste	Mushrooms, shiitake	Potatoes	Water chestnuts
Chili flakes	Mushrooms, variety	Potatoes, red skin	Watercress
Chilies, green	Mustard, honey	Potatoes, sweet	Wine, burgundy
Cilantro	Mustard	Prunes	Wine, white
Cinnamon	Nutmeg	Raisins	Wintergreen
Coriander	Oil, olive	Rice, brown	Worcester sauce
Corn	Oil, peanut	Rice, white	Yogurt
Cranberry	Oil, safflower	Rose Hips	Zucchini
Cucumber	Oil, sesame	Rosemary	
Cumin	Oil, walnut	Saffron	

LYCOPENE:
Nature's Miraculous Cell Defender

Of the 20 or so carotenoids that regularly occur in blood plasma, only one has the rare ability to impede disease-causing reactions at the fastest rate. Lycopene, which is the principle red pigment present in apricots, tomatoes, guava, watermelon, paprika, pink grapefruit, rose hips, and palm oil, owns this "title.". The table to the right lists the amounts of Lycopene found in some fruits and vegetables.

Similar chemically to Beta-Carotene, this remarkable carotenoid supersedes all others in its singlet oxygen quenching efficiency. In fact, it exhibits the highest overall quenching capacity of all carotenoids. The calculated quenching rate constant (Kq) for Lycopene was more than double that of Beta-Carotene.

Now, not all carotenoids have the same antioxidant potential. Some quench free radicals more ably than others. Of the 20 or so carotenoids that regularly occur in blood plasma, a ranking of free-radical or singlet oxygen quenching rates have been studied in *in vitro* conditions. Among the carotenoids several supersede Beta-Carotene in their singlet oxygen quenching efficiency, with Lycopene exhibiting the highest overall quenching capacity. The calculated quenching rate constant (Kq) for Lycopene was more than double that of Beta-Carotene. Lycopene, found in abundance in tomatoes, is also found in palm oil.

Of the common carotenoids present in foods, Lycopene was found to be particularly active against carcinogenesis. It was inversely associated with cancers of the pancreas and cervix in analysis of human blood level studies. Interestingly, individual carotenoids seem to be absorbed in differing quantities by individual organs. This further supports the concept that we should consume a variety of carotenoids for the broadest range of protection.

This vital cell protector has been known for some time. Commercial development of Lycopene was delayed until recently because the amount contained in tomatoes

Lycopene Content of Selected Fruits and Vegetables
(in micrograms per 100 grams)

Apricot	65	ug/100 g
Apricot, dried	864	
Apricot, raw	5	
Grapefruit, pink & raw	3,362	
Guava juice	3,340	
Rose hip puree	780	
Tomato juice, canned	8,580	
Tomato paste, canned	6,500	
Tomato sauce, canned	6,300	
Watermelon, raw	4,100	

was found to be too low to make extraction commercially feasible. To solve this problem and bring concentrated quantities of Lycopene to the consumer at a reasonable cost, an Israel-based chemical company launched an ambitious program spanning years. Intensive research and development involving the efforts of scientists, engineers, and food technologists resulted in new tomato varieties with a Lycopene content 4-5 times higher than that found in average edible tomatoes. The extracted Lycopene (and other carotenoids) has been shown as surviving intact from the extraction and processing procedures. Most importantly, no chemical reactions are involved in producing this trade-marked brand named Lyc-O-Pen. Standardized to 5% Lycopene, this is a natural tomato product.

ALPHA AND BETA-CAROTENE (Carotenoids)

You have no doubt heard and read about the health benefits of Beta-Carotene. *Over 70 studies conducted worldwide show that people lower their risk for cancer if they eat sufficient amounts of carotenoids.* Epidemiological evidence supports the premise that the *carotenoids offer protection against certain types of cancer due to their antioxidant activity.* Yet only recently has the scientific community and general public recognized the relationship of free radicals and antioxidants to health. Free radicals are unstable molecules with unpaired electrons that damage cell membranes and cause cell mutations. Antioxidants inhibit free radicals. This intensive view of inner cellular warfare may hold the keys to protecting humankind against premature aging and the associated diseases of aging.

Let us now focus on that remarkable class of compounds—the carotenoids— and see how some of them are more equal than others when it comes to cellular defense as it relates to antioxidant activity.

WHAT ARE CAROTENOIDS?

The carotenoids trap sunlight so that green plants can conduct photosynthesis. Remember, the collection of the sun's energy by green plants and the conversion of carbon dioxide and water into glucose is the basis for life on earth! So to understand the carotenoids is to grasp the miracle and meaning of existence.

Technically carotenoids are classified as 40 carbon tetraterpenoids, but to the unaided eye they are the compounds that provide the brilliant colors found in nature. In flowers this rainbow of compounds mainly appear as yellow colors (as in daffodils, pansy, sunflowers); in fruit they project a red or orange color (rose hip, tomato, paprika, acerola, red pepper).

Carotenes were first discovered in 1831 in carrots, hence the name. There are now 563 known carotenoids. Of these, about 50 can be metabolized to Vitamin A (Retinole) by many animals. This conversion to vitamin A was once thought to be of importance only to nutritionists until the recent discoveries of the carotenes' antioxidant properties.

HOW DO CAROTENOIDS ACT TO PROTECT OUR CELLS?

The carotenoids are readily oxidized (they *lose* or give up electrons) and so limit *other* oxidation reactions within cells. That is, the carotenoids figuratively *"sacrifice themselves"* in the oxygen wars so our cells may live!

Newer evidence shows that carotenoids not only act as *passive* players in the oxygen wars, but they also function *actively* as antioxidants by quenching various free-radicals that are generated inside cells. This occurs when excitation energy is transferred from the highly reactive singlet oxygen ($^1O_2$) to the carotenoid:

$$^1O_2 \; + \; \text{carotenoid} \; \longrightarrow \; ^3O_2 \; + \; ^3\text{carotenoid}$$

(singlet oxygen) (triplet oxygen) (carotenoid triplet)

In a subsequent reaction, the excitation energy is harmlessly dissipated:

$$^3\text{carotenoid} \; \longrightarrow \; \text{carotenoid} + \text{heat} \quad \text{(from Krinsky, 1989)}$$

In this sequence of reactions a carotenoid acts similarly to a catalyst to neutralize the highly reactive singlet oxygen molecule by functioning as an antioxidant.

ALPHA AND BETA CAROTENE

Newer evidence now shows that some carotenoids, especially Alpha- Carotene, have remarkable antioxidant activities. While Beta-Carotene generates vitamin A twice as efficiently as Alpha-Carotene, Alpha-Carotene is approximately ten times more powerful in inhibiting skin, lung, and liver carcinogenesis. The carotenoids may have highly specialized physiological functions, which may explain why Alpha-Carotene has been associated with lower cancer mortality in epidemiological studies, as well as anti-carcinogenic effects in animal studies.

In fact, one of the world's leading cancer researchers, Dr. M. Murakoshi, has shown that Alpha-Carotene obtained from palm oil is more protective against carcinogens than Beta-Carotene. Indeed, Murakoshi found that the carotenes inhibited already present cancerous growths from further growths, particularly liver cancer.

The role of Alpha-Carotene in the quenching of singlet oxygen in blood plasma indicates this remarkable yet little known carotenoid can *protect* low density lipoprotein (LDL) from oxidation and *thereby reduce the risk of heart attacks from arteriosclerosis and myocardial ischemia.*

A very recent multicenter case-control study in nine European countries further supports this trend of medical reasoning. In a study of 683 people with acute myocardial infarction (MI or heart attack) and 727 people without a history of this disease, researchers found that the higher amounts of antioxidants in fat tissue reduce the risk of a first heart attack. *In particular, high Beta-Carotene levels were found to be the most protective of the antioxidants studied.* Low tissues levels of Beta-Carotene in smokers greatly increased the risk of MI, which suggests a relationship between oxidative stress, aging and many diseases, including heart attack. Other health benefits from alpha and Beta-Carotene may include a reduced risk of cataract.

Further evidence of the specialized nature of the carotenoids is demonstrated by the appearance of two carotenoids in the macular region of the retina where Beta-Carotene is totally absent. These two retina specific carotenoids are *Zeaxanthin* (a yellow pigment found in corn seeds, sweet red pepper, bitter orange peel, and in green algae) and *Lutein* (found in the green leaves of all higher plants, also in algae, in citrus rind, in apricot, peach, plum, apple, and cranberry).

HOW THE ANTIOXIDANTS COMPLEMENT RATHER THAN COMPETE WITH ONE ANOTHER

Interestingly, just as foods work together so do the antioxidants. Professor Lester Packer of the University of California at Berkeley is one of the world's pre-eminent antioxidant researchers. He and coworkers recently demonstrated how carotenoids interact with vitamins E and C. Beta-Carotene, it was shown, can protect LDL against oxidative damage even when vitamin E levels are low.

This is a variation on the old theme among nutritionists to "eat a wide variety of foods." But it makes good sense because if we do eat widely of fruits and vegetables we gain from nature's pharmacy her many protective substances, especially the carotenoids and flavonoids. Currently there is not a Recommended Daily Allowance (RDA) for carotenes. However the NCI (National Cancer Institute) guide recommends 6 mg of Beta-Carotene per day and some researchers believe the daily intake should be as high as 15 to 20 mg. Average daily consumption in the U.S. is 1.5 mg (according to U.S.D.A. studies). Now it is also true that we rarely eat consistently wisely, especially when we are busy and when we travel, which is why we take and recommend nutrients and other supplements.

THE BEST IN NATURE

As the science of nutrition unfolds the secrets of nature we are discovering how nature was meant to be taken whole. Whole grains but not refined grains, for example, give us all the vitamin E and the full B complex found in nature. For years we have known about the numerous health benefits of Beta-Carotene. We now know that a range of carotenoids, including Alpha-Carotene and Lycopene, give us the best means of enhancing our natural defenses. We are not talking about discarding or ignoring all of medical history, but about using as many of the natural nutrients as possible to enhance and strengthen our ability to resist illness and degenerative disease, using this knowledge in conjunction with the developments of modern science.

Lately, phytochemical research has greatly intensified and we are pleased to say that our recipes are all confirmed by the experts. In conclusion, we are reprintings in its entirety the following paper by Dr. Weiner, *Herbal Antioxidants in Clinical Practice*, presented in the summer of 1994 at the Linus Pauling Institute Conference held at Tiburon, California. We hope you enjoy cooking with Superfoods!

HERBAL ANTIOXIDANTS IN CLINICAL PRACTICE

Antioxidant. The word itself is magic. Suggesting some type of all-encompassing protection against cellular wear and damage, the scientific-medical community has now embraced a once reviled theory. Using the antioxidant concept as a spearhead in proposed mechanisms for staving off so-called "free- radical" reactions, the rush is on to mine claims for the latest and most effective combination of free-radical scavenging compounds.

Without disputing or supporting the concept that aggressive oxygen species are the new culprit for most illnesses (superseding the microbial causative drama of the 19th century), we must acknowledge that such "radicals" have definitively been shown to damage all biochemical components such as DNA/RNA; carbohydrates; unsaturated lipids; proteins; and micronutrients such as carotenoids (Alpha and Beta Carotene, Lycopene), vitamins A, B6, B12, and folate.

Defense strategies against such aggressive radical species include enzymes, antioxidants that occur naturally in the body (glutathione, uric acid, ubiquinol-10, and others) and radical scavenging nutrients, such as vitamins A, C, and E, and carotenoids.

This paper will present a brief discussion of some well- and little-known phytopharmaceuticals (i.e., herbs) that may add to the optimization of antioxidant status and therefore offer added preventive values for overall health.

It is important to state at the outset that antioxidants vary widely in their free-radical quenching effects and each may be individually attracted to specific cell sites. Further evidence of the specialized nature of the carotenoids is demonstrated by the appearance of two carotenoids in the macular region of the retina where Beta-Carotene is totally absent. These two retina specific carotenoids are *zeaxanthin* (a yellow pigment found in corn seeds, sweet red pepper, bitter orange peel, and in green algae) and *Lutein* (found in the green leaves of all higher plants, also in algae, in citrus rind, in apricot, peach, plum, apple, and cranberry).

As scientific inquiry proceeds we will likely learn of other site-specific attractions and functions of the carotenoids. This will help us understand why we need not reject one class of antioxidant compounds to accept another. They each may accumulate in specialized cells and tissues, with some overlapping protection, but a variety of them is required to give us the best protection possible.

As we have noted, just as foods work together so do the antioxidants. Dr. Packer and coworkers recently demonstrated how carotenoids interact with vitamins E and C. Beta-Carotene, it was shown, can protect LDL against oxidative damage even when vitamin E levels are low.

In this regard, antioxidants act synergistically, offering a rainbow of protection rather than a single band of the spectrum. Moreover, plant antioxidants such as phenols and bioflavonoids may potentiate vitamin antioxidants. For example, rutin, a bioflavonoid, potentiates vitamins C and E when taken in combination, yielding a *more potent* radical scavenging action. That is, adding a *third* antioxidant (rutin) creates a combined effect greater than the sum of the parts.

SOME MAJOR ANTIOXIDANT HERBS

Antioxidant factors found in plants are based upon constituent nutrients with demonstrated radical-scavenging capacities as well as upon non-vitamin or mineral substances. So, in addition to alpha-tocopherol, ascorbate, carotenoids, and zinc, plant-based medicines may contain flavonoids, polyphenols, and flavoproteins. Further, some plants or specific combinations of herbs in formulations may act as antioxidants by exerting superoxide scavenging activity or by increasing superoxide dismutase (SOD) activity in various tissue sites. Each of these groups of compounds are substances that may exert that cell-protective action by more than one biochemical mechanism.

In addition to antioxidant properties *per se*, cancer-protective factors are found in many plants, including some fruits, vegetables, and commonly used spices and herbs.

They can be divided into several different groups, based on their chemical structure, e.g., polyphenols, thiols, carotenoids and retinoids, carbohydrates, trace metals, terpenes, tocopherols and degradation products of glucosinolates (i.e., isothiocyanates, indoles and dithiothiols) and others. Among each of these groups of compounds are substances, which may exert their cancer-protective action by more than one biochemical mechanism. The biochemical processes of carcinogenesis are still not known in detail and probably varies with the cancer disease in question. Accordingly, the description of the biochemical backgrounds for the actions of cancer-protective factors must be based on a simplified model of the process of carcinogenesis. The model used in this presentation is a generalized initiation-promotion-conversion model, in which initiators are thought to be directly or indirectly genotoxic, promoters are visualized as substances capable of inferring a growth advantage on initiated cells and converters are believed to be genotoxic, e.g. mutagens, clastogens, recombinogens or the like. Experimental evidence for the mechanisms of action of cancer-protective agents in fruits and vegetables that protect against initiation include the scavenging effects of polyphenols on activated mutagens and carcinogens, the quenching of singlet oxygen and radicals by carotenoids, the antioxidant effects of many compounds including ascorbic acid and polyphenols, the inhibition of activating enzymes by some flavonols and tannins, the induction of oxidation and of conjugation (protective) enzymes by indoles, isothiocyanates and dithiothiones, the shielding of sensitive structures by some polyphenols and the stimulation of DNA-repair exerted by sulphur-containing compounds. Mechanisms at the biochemical level in antipromotion include the antioxidant effects of carotenoids and the membrane stabilizing effects reported with polyphenols, the inhibition of proteases caused by compounds from soybeans, the stimulation of immune responses seen with carotenoids and ascorbic acid, and the inhibition of ornithine decarboxylase by polyphenols and carotenoids. A few inhibitors of conversion have been identified experimentally, and it can be argued on a theoretical basis, that many inhibitors of initiation should also be efficient against conversion. The mechanisms of anticarcinogenic substances in fruits and vegetables are discussed in the light of cancer prevention and inhibition.

Plant antioxidants are more than mere supporting players in the battle against cellular damage and disease. As folklore has long instructed, certain plants play specific roles in disease prevention and treatment. A well known hepatic antioxidant, *silymarin*, from the milk thistle (*Silybum marianum*), for example, inhibits liver damage by scavenging free radicals among other mechanisms. This powerful antioxidant protects the liver against alcohol and pharmaceutical injury and even poisoning from extremely toxic compounds found in the Deathcap mushroom, *Amanita phalloides*. Interestingly, the *Amanita* toxins are *not* thought to be neutralized via any free-radical scavenging effects. Rather, it is theorized that silymarin competes with the *Amanita* toxins for the identical receptor on cell membranes. Here again, contemporary laboratory science confirms and elucidates the liver-protecting attributes of milk thistle, well known to folk medicine for 2,000 years.

CAYENNE

Scientific Name: *Capsicum frutescens*
Parts Used: Fruit
Dosage: Fruit: 1/4 to 1 whole teaspoon per cup of hot water.

Recent Scientific Findings

Cayenne pepper acts as a rubefacient when applied externally, and as a stimulant internally, due to the presence of *capsaicin,* which is the "hot principle" in the fruits of this plant. Oleoresin of *Capsicum* is still used in the preparation of a number of popular proprietary products to be applied locally for the relief of sore muscles, and produces the desired effect by mildly irritating the surface of the skin, which causes an increased blood flow to the area of application. The increased blood flow reduces inflammation of the affected area.

Capsaicin, a phenol present in Cayenne pepper, has shown a variety of medicinal benefits. In a recent letter to *The Lancet*, it was reported that topical applications of capsaicin cream completely alleviated the severe stump pain experienced by a middle-aged female diabetic. This double-amputee patient subsequently underwent a placebo trial, where it was proved that while this cream completely relieved the pain, the placebo having no effect. Given the successful outcome of this extreme example, it would be reasonable to expect capsaicin creams to yield beneficial topical results when applied to various painful neuropathies.

Further information regarding the anti-inflammatory property of capsaicin is revealed in the paper, "Direct Evidence for Neurogenic Inflammation and its Prevention by Denervation and by Pretreatment with Capsaicin," as quoted in Dr. Garcia-Leme's book, *Hormones and Inflammation,* 1989. In studies with rats given capsaicin systemically, the results proved, "sensory nerve endings became insensitive to chemical pain stimuli for a long time. Neurogenic inflammation cannot be elicited in animals pretreated with capsaicin."

Additionally, two Indian scientists recently reported that long-term treatment with capsaicin "desensitizes" the membrane against various gaseous irritant-induced free radical damage. They found that this compound protects lung tissue (in experiments with rats) by increasing superoxide dismutase (SOD), catalase (CAT) and peroxidase (POD) activities. In as yet unpublished studies by the same authors, pretreatment with capsaicin also protected the lung of rats from nitrogen dioxide and formaldehyde induced free radical damage.

Two double-blind studies with human patients investigated a capsaicin-based pharmaceutical's effect on the daily activities of patients suffering from the nerve pain associated with diabetes. Such neuropathy usually interferes with the ability to work, sleep, walk, eat, use shoes and socks, and enjoy recreational activities. This complication of diabetes often upsets and reduces the overall quality of a patient's life, the pain usually lasting for many years.

The failure of drugs such as tricyclic antidepressants, anticonvulsants, narcotic analgesics, and phenothiazines for this condition has led to the search for safer, more effective alternatives. The medical world has found that nature has succeeded where synthesis has failed.

Researchers at the prestigious Scripps Clinic and Research Foundation in La Jolla, California, enrolled 277 men and women with this painful condition (nerve pain) and followed them for 8 weeks in this double-blind study. The capcaicin cream was tried against a neutral cream and applied to the painful areas four times daily. Statistically significant differences were observed, with improvement in favor of the capsaicin cream. Such a natural-based medicine is now being utilized to improve the lives of thousands.

The marvelous benefits of capsaicin were reported earlier by a group from Henry Ford Hospital in Detroit, Michigan. This double-blind study tested 15 patients with diabetes mellitus suffering from neuropathy. The authors concluded that this plant-derived compound is "potentially effective when burning pain is a major symptom of PDN. The side effects of capsaicin were limited and minimal. This agent should be considered by clinicians for treatment of PDN."

Also human studies have been done on Capsaicin's effectiveness in treating rhinitis. The drug was given to patients three times daily for three days. The patients' symptoms were recorded over a one month period. The results indicated that the Capsaicin treatment markedly reduced nasal obstruction and nasal secretion.

Interestingly, both cayenne pepper preparations and the active principle *capsaicin* have been shown in humans and in animals to stimulate the production of gastric juices, resulting in improved digestion.

CITRUS

Scientific Name: Various species
Parts Used: Essential oils extracted from peel of lemons and oranges
Dosage: 1 to 5 capsules, 2 to 3 times per day.

Recent Scientific Findings

In recent years, research has uncovered anti-cancer properties in certain essential oils. Limonene is the major component of the essential oil of orange and other citrus fruits. It also occurs widely in the plant kingdom, particularly in those species producing essential oils, flavors and spices. This compound belongs to a class of natural compounds known as terpenes, soon to equal the bioflavonoids and carotenoids in their applications.

About ten animal studies have been published which show that dietary limonene (the d-isomer, or d-limonene) lowers the incidence of chemically-induced cancers as well as delaying their appearance. Elson and colleagues at the University of Wisconsin are currently the leaders in this field. In one study, they demonstrated that dietary d-limonene markedly reduced dimethylbenzanthracene-induced mammary cancers. The dosage used in this study was 1000 parts per million, or 1 gram per kg of diet. [NOTE: humans eat about 1/2 kg per day, which translates to about 500 mg of d-limonene per day.]

Using this same model system, they subsequently showed that the essential oil of orange (85% d-limonene) was more effective than pure d-limonene in preventing tumor formation. Thus, naturally-occurring terpenes in orange oil other than d-limonenes also possess anticancer activity. Further investigations by this group revealed that dietary d-limonene is effective in reversing preformed tumors, as evidenced by an increase in the tumor regression rate. Finally, Elson and associates recently observed that dietary d-limonene was effective in reducing the number of chemically-induced mammary tumors in rats when provided either during the initiation phase or during the promotion/progression phase.

The mechanism(s) of action of d-limonene against cancer are not well understood, but may involve the enhancement of drug-metabolizing systems such as *glutathione-S-transferases*. The ability of d-limonene to reverse preformed tumors and to inhibit tumor growth during the promotion/progression phase of cancer suggests an immunostimulating action, and some recent evidence does support this concept.

As an added benefit limonene is a potent, natural cholesterol-lowering compound. It acts by inhibiting the same enzyme (HMG-coenzyme A reductase) which is the target of many prescribed cholesterol-reducing drugs such as lovostatin. If these actions were not sufficient, limonene is also a powerful agent for dissolving gallstones.

Researchers at the University of Wisconsin, Madison, confirmed d-limonene's antitumor potential. In a series of animal experiments, up to 90% of tumors completely disappeared in mice fed this compound, whereas only 15% of tumors spontaneously diminished in size in animals not given the compound. Human cancer cells have also been shrunk with d-limonene in laboratory experiments. Michael Gould, professor of human oncology at the University of Wisconsin was quoted as saying "we can potentially use limonene to treat as well as prevent cancer."

In another study of d-limonene it was found that gallstones were dissolved by this "simple, safe, and effective solvent."

GARLIC

Scientific Name: *Allium sativum*
Parts Used: Cloves
Dosage: 1/2 teaspoon of the juice 3 times daily

Recent Scientific Findings

As knowledge about the benefits of Garlic continues to spread from folklore into mainstream medicine, numerous claims are being made regarding various Garlic products. Before looking at some of these claims we should summarize the health significance of Garlic and Garlic constituents.

One of the world's leading authorities on this subject is Dr. Eric Block, a professor of chemistry at the State University of New York at Albany. His review article published in *Scientific American* remains an important summary of the chemistry of this fascinating plant.

To summarize, here are some of the claimed nutritional and pharmacological properties of Garlic:

1. Lowers serum total and low density lipoprotein cholesterol in humans.

2. Raises high density lipoprotein cholesterol (HDL's), in humans.

3. Reduces the tendency of blood to clot, and the aggregation (i.e. clumping) of blood platelets.

4. Inhibits inflammation by modulating the conversion of arachidonic acid (A.A.) to eicosanids.

5. Inhibits cancer cell formation and proliferation by inhibiting nitrosamine formation, modulating the metabolism of polyarene carcinogens, and acting on cell enzymes which control cell division.

6. Protects the liver from damage induced by synthetic drugs and chemical pollutants.

7. Kills intestinal parasites and worms, as well as gram-negative bacteria.

8. Protects against the effects of radiation.

9. Offers antioxidant protection to cell membranes.

Some of these health effects are worth looking at in more detail. Perhaps most significant is the effect of Garlic and onion and their extracts on the lipid profile of blood and tissues. They lower cholesterol, triglycerides and LDL cholesterol levels while also increasing the beneficial cholesterol, HDL.

Both Garlic and onion oils inhibit the enzymes lipoxygenase and cyclooxygenase. Each of these enzymes is known to act on one of two parallel biochemical pathways (within the arachidonic acid cascade) and only by inhibiting these enzymes can this pathway be arrested. When arrested, the production of prostaglandin is slowed. Since many cancers are prostaglandin dependent, this may explain why the *allium* oils have antitumor properties.

Garlic and onion contain over 75 different sulfur-containing compounds. While most of the medical benefits derived from supplementation with extracts of these plants are a result of these sulfurous compounds, recent studies show the additional presence of the bioflavonoids quercitin and cyanidin.

The cellular antioxidant Selenium is another constituent found in the *allium* vegetables and their extracts. The antitumor effects claimed for selenium may be based on its ability to replace the sulphur in the amino acid l-cystine. Leukemic white blood cells have a rapid turnover of l-cystine, a similar amino acid, and by substituting selenium for sulphur, leukemia can be suppressed, in animals.

Recent research in China demonstrated a significant inverse relationship between the incidence of stomach cancer and the intake of Garlic and related *allium* vegetables. The researchers interviewed 1131 controls and 564 patients with stomach cancer and found that people with no stomach cancer ate significantly higher amounts of *allium* vegetables (a mean intake of 19.0 kg/year) than did the cancer patients (a mean intake of 15.5 kg/year). Those people who ate less than 11.5 kg/year were more than twice as likely to develop stomach cancer than were people who ate more than 24 kg/year.

Researchers at the Garlic Research Bureau in Suffolk, England, recently found "that even small amounts of Garlic, say 3 or 4 grams, will have a pronounced effect on fibrinolytic activity . . . in doses from 25 grams (10 cloves) to 50 grams Garlic seems to be highly effective in promoting beneficial changes in blood fat composition and in platelet adhesiveness."

To understand which type of Garlic—the raw, the cooked, or the preserved—may be most beneficial, we must look at the chemical changes which occur inside a Garlic clove. Fresh whole Garlic is pharmacologically inactive. When crushed, an internal enzyme acts on *alliin,* a sulphur-containing amino acid, to produce the reactive compound known as *allicin.* Left to stand in the air or when cooked, allicin is destroyed.

While there is no final scientific agreement on the therapeutically active component of Garlic, there is a consensus that allicin is very important, both as an active component itself or as a precursor of other active components. Because it is unstable, it has been difficult to manufacture a Garlic product with significant amounts of allicin. The term "allicin potential" has been created to refer to the established standard of activity found in fresh Garlic. Obviously, fresh Garlic is highly desirable, for those who can tolerate the strong taste and aroma.

To receive Garlic's benefits without consuming cloves and cloves each day, utilize the product form. The minimum effective dosage for benefiting the cardiovascular system is one clove (3 grams of fresh or 1 gram of dried) per day. Obviously, more would increase these benefits.

To prevent the pungent odor from seeping out in the breath some manufacturers are utilizing enteric coating. This moves the breakdown of alliin and alynase from the stomach to the small intestine.

GINGER

Scientific Name: *Zingiber officinale*
Parts Used: Rhizome
Dosage: Root: 1 ounce of rhizome to 1 pint of water. Boil the water separately, then pour over the plant material and steep for 5 to 20 minutes, depending on the desired effect. Drink hot or warm, 1 to 2 cups per day.

Recent Scientific Findings

Currently, Ginger has received new attention as an aid to prevent nausea from motion sickness. Ginger tea has long been an American herbal remedy for coughs and asthma, related to allergy or inflammation; the creation of the soft drink ginger ale, sprang from the common folkloric usage of this herb, and still today remains a popular beverage for the relief of stomach upset. Externally, Ginger is a rubefacient, and has been credited in this connection with relieving headache and toothache.

The mechanism by which Ginger produces anti-inflammatory activity is that of the typical NSAID (non-steroidal anti-inflammatory drug). This common spice is a more biologically active prostaglandin inhibitor (via cyclo-oxygenase inhibition) than onion and Garlic.

By slowing associated biochemical pathways an inflammatory reaction is curtailed. In one study, Danish women between the ages of 25 to 65 years, consumed either 70 grams raw onion or 5 grams raw ginger daily for a period of one week. The author measured thromboxane production and discovered that ginger, more clearly than onion, reduced thromboxane production by almost 60%. This confirms the Ayurvedic "prescription" for this common spice and its anti-aggregatory effects.

By reducing blood platelet "clumping," Ginger, Onion and Garlic may reduce our risk of heart attack or stroke. In a series of experiments with rats, scientists from Japan discovered that extracts of Ginger inhibited gastric lesions by up to 97%. The authors conclude that the folkloric usage of Ginger in stomachic preparations were effective owing to the constituents zingiberene, the main terpenoid and 6-gingerol, the pungent principle.

In an earlier look at how some of the active components of Ginger (and onion) act inside our cells, it was found that the oils of these herbs inhibit the fatty acid oxygenases from platelets, thus decreasing the clumping of these blood cell components.

A 1991 double-blind, randomized cross-over trial involved thirty women suffering from hyperemesis gravidarum. Ginger was alternated with a placebo. Seventy percent of the women confirmed they subjectively preferred the period in which they took the Ginger. More objective assessment verified the subjective reactions, as significantly greater relief was found after the use of the Ginger.

In a series of experiments with rats, scientists from Japan discovered that extracts of ginger inhibited gastric lesions by up to 97%. The authors concluded that the folkloric usage of Ginger in stomachic preparations was effective due to the constituents zingiberene, the main terpenoid, and 6-gingerol, the pungent principle.

GINSENG, SIBERIAN

Scientific Name: *Eleutherococcus senticosus*
Parts Used: Root
Dosage: Powder: 1/2 teaspoon of powder to 1 cup of hot water. Drink in the morning, at lunch, at bedtime (add Lemongrass if you find the flavor wanting).

Recent Scientific Findings

Traditionally touted for its "aphrodisiac" effect, many people are under the impression that Ginseng is only a "male" herb. In actuality, the Siberian Ginseng is highly valued by both sexes for its adaptogenic abilities. An adaptogen is a substance that "normalizes" adverse conditions of the body.

Ginseng has always been perceived as a stimulant. In Russia a great deal of publicity comes from its use by cosmonauts and Olympic athletes to provide energy and negate stress effects. Most remarkably, victims of the Chernobyl nuclear disaster were given courses of *Eleutherococcus* to aid them with an anti-radiation effect. Russians prescribe Siberian Ginseng for patients undergoing chemotherapy and radiotherapy.

While the chemical constituents, "eleutherosides," differ from those of *Panax* species, the pharmacological effects of Siberian Ginseng are quite similar to those of *Panax ginseng*. This plant has been studied more rigorously by the Russians than *Panax ginseng*; they have studied both species, in fact. Extracts of Siberian Ginseng have been shown to relieve stress, lower the toxicity of some common drugs that tend to produce side effects in humans, increase mental alertness, improve resistance to colds and mild infections, and be beneficial in cases where a person is continuously in contact with environmental stresses.

A recent (1987) first-rate double-blind study demonstrated that a Siberian Ginseng extract stimulated cellular immunity. Thirty-six healthy volunteers received 10 milliliters of an alcohol extract of Siberian Ginseng three times daily for four weeks. A placebo of plain ethanol was used. A "drastic increase in the absolute number of [immune] cells," especially T lymphocytes was shown using flow cytometry. The T helper/inducer cells, as well as cytotoxic and natural killer cells were increased in number, which is clear demonstration that the human immune system can be augmented with this herb. As expected, no side effects were observed during the experiment or afterwards, a period of six months.

Flow cytometry is a highly advanced means for observing cells that permits an analysis of individual living cells. Using this method to study human immune reactions, German researchers proved that an extract of Siberian Ginseng stimulated T cell production, especially helper cells. This proof that such an "adaptogen" truly works pushes herbal science into mainstream medicine with wide application in numerous immune-related disorders.

The German scientists stated Siberian Ginseng "could be considered a nonspecific immunostimulant." This may help explain why it has been said to be of benefit or cited in "protective effects against viral infections, retardation of neoplastic growth and metastasis, or better tolerance of chemotherapy and radiation." They further speculated "about a positive effect of *eleutherococcus* in very early stages of HIV (AIDS) infection by preventing or retarding the spread of the virus, mediated by a synergistic action of elevated numbers of both helper and cytotoxic T cells."

It is not likely that any of the eleutherosides or ginsenosides will ever be used as adaptogens by themselves, since they are only present in their respective plants in small amounts. Similarly, they are too complex to expect a commercially feasible synthesis. Professor I. I. Brekhman, who has conducted numerous animal and human experiments with both *Panax ginseng* and *Eleutherococcus senticosus*, claims that the adaptogenic effect requires the total mixture of eleutherosides, in the case of Siberian Ginseng at least, and that the full effects cannot be obtained with any one of the pure eleutherosides.

Unlike *Panax ginseng, Eleutherococcus senticosus* does not seem to cause insomnia, and like *Panax ginseng,* there do not appear to be any adverse effects in humans from the use of Siberian Ginseng.

GREEN TEA

Scientific Name: Various spp.
Parts Used: Leaves
Dosage: Leaves: Approximately 1 ounce of leaves to 1 pint of water. Boil water separately and pour over the plant material and steep for 5 to 20 minutes, depending on the desired effect. Drink hot or warm, 1 to 2 cups per day, at bedtime and upon awakening.

Recent Scientific Findings

Modern scientists are discovering new healthful benefits from the consumption of Green Tea. According to Hirota Fujiki, a chemist at the National Cancer Center Research Institute in Tokyo, "This Green Tea cannot prevent every cancer, but it's the cheapest and most practical method for cancer prevention available to the general public."

The majority of teas produced worldwide can be classified into two types: black tea, which is most common in Western nations, and Green Tea, which predominates in the Far East, especially China and Japan. When consumed, Green Tea provides more healthful advantages than black tea because it contains larger amounts of such important substances as vitamins, including twice as much vitamin C as black tea.

Green Tea contains more than twice the catechins of black tea; tea's "tannins" consist mostly of these catechins. Though the content of vitamin P in other foods is very low, tea catechins have been found to have high vitamin P activity. In fact, the regular consumption of catechin-rich tea may meet the human requirements for vitamin P, according to some researchers.

While tea's favorable effect was once attributed to its caffeine content, biochemical studies have shown that tea's catechins may play an even greater role. It has been demonstrated that peculiar features of the chemical composition of tea are responsible for its important pharmacological and physiological properties. Tea's beneficial effects that were first discovered empirically over many generations have been corroborated by present-day scientific investigations.

The catechins in tea are formed by polyphenic compounds. Many researchers have found that phenolic compounds, including tea catechins, delay the development of arteriosclerosis. Clinical investigations ascertained that consumption of Green Tea had a therapeutic effect on infectious diseases, particularly dysentery. Incorporating Green Tea in the treatment of rheumatism had a favorable effect on both the general condition and capillary resistance of their patients. The researchers concluded that Green Tea exerts a favorable regulatory effect on every vital component of human metabolism.

Green Tea polyphols, which comprise from 17-30% of the dry weight of Green Tea leaves, are now known to explain the panacea-like properties of the world's most popular beverage. Found recently to account for the anti-viral, antioxidant effects in Green Tea, these unique polyphenols also enhance immunity and destroy bacteria. Epidemiological surveys suggest that Green Tea consumption is associated with a reduced incidence of pancreatic and stomach cancers.

In recent years there has been a growing interest in identifying the antimutagenic and anticarcinogenic constituents of the human diet. Here again, researchers are discovering that Green Tea provides healthful benefits. From a series of mouse experiments Wang and his colleagues concluded, "These results, in conjunction with our prior publications, suggest that consumption of Green Tea may reduce the risk of some forms of human cancer induced by both physical and chemical environmental carcinogens."

At the Fourth Chemical Congress of North America, Japanese and U.S. researchers reported that Green Tea helps shield mice against tumors of the liver, lung, skin, and digestive tract and may do the same for humans. In 1987, epigallocatechin gallate (EGCG) was found to be the key protective ingredient. EBCG seems to possess the broadest spectrum and level of activity of the Green Tea polyphenols and makes up more than 50% of the total GTP content. Researchers speculated that this antioxidant may protect against tumor development by destroying free radicals (highly reactive atoms or molecules) that could otherwise attack DNA and disrupt normal cell processes. In mice given a carcinogen that affects the digestive tract, 20 percent of the animals treated with EGCG developed intestinal cancer compared with 63% that did not get EGCG.

At the same time, EGCG may prevent the activation of certain carcinogens so that free radicals never form. Researchers at Rutgers University reported similar findings regarding skin cancer. The incidence of skin cancer is steadily increasing and the disease represents a major health and economic problem in the modern industrialized world. Mice that drank Green Tea instead of plain water for 10 days before and during exposure to ultraviolet light proved less susceptible to skin damage. "These broad effects of the Green Tea are quite interesting. There aren't that many things that have as broad a spectrum," mused study director Allan H. Conney. Much research remains to be done in this area, however. "The results are encouraging, but I think it would be premature to extrapolate these studies to humans," said Conney. It is not yet known how well the mouse data may apply to humans.

Currently, the speculation of Green Tea's cancer inhibiting effects in humans is based on demographic extrapolations. It has been surmised that Green Tea may explain why Japanese cigarette smokers have a lower rate of lung cancer than smokers in the United States. People residing in Shizuoka, Japan's tea-growing region, use tea leaves only once instead of as in other areas of Japan where the same leaves are used several times. Therefore, the people of Shizuoka consume greater quantities of the tea's chemicals. In Shizuoka the death rate from cancer, especially stomach cancer, is markedly lower than in the rest of Japan. Significant differences for habitual Green Tea consumption between Nakakawane City and Osuka City were observed. In Osuka, people drink less tea and have a high mortality rate due to stomach cancer. In Nakakawane, people drink more tea and have a low rate of stomach cancer.

Green Tea also stabilizes blood lipids, and may therefore be of value in an overall cardiac-care regimen. According to a 1991 study on mice, Green Tea extract prevented an increase in serum cholesterol even when the animals were fed an atherogenic (i.e., artery-damaging) diet. Serum lipid peroxides were also diminished, while the destruction of lecithin was reduced.

An antioxidant fraction of Green Tea Extract has been shown to efficiently scavenge the pro-oxidants hydrogen peroxide and superoxide anion radical, and to protect against the cytotoxicity of paraquat, a biocide that exhibits cellular toxicity via a pro-oxidant intermediate. Studies evaluating the ability of various polyphenols and condensed tannins (procyanidins linked to gallic acid) to scavenge the various pro-oxidants revealed that EGCG was the most potent; EGCG was also most effective at inhibiting lipid peroxidation in brain tissues from animals, exhibiting over 200 times greater activity than vitamin E (alpha-tocopherol). These investigators postulated that the galloyl groups may lend themselves to increasing antioxidant effectiveness.

EGCG and Epicatechin Gallate have recently been shown to selectively inhibit reverse transcriptase in Human Immunodeficiency Virus (HIV-RT), whereas the constituent building blocks of these compounds had no inhibitory activity. The most attractive feature of these results rests upon the observation that inhibition of HIV-RT was observed at gallocatechin concentrations over 5 times less than that which inhibited "normal" cellular DNA polymerases. This is a promising finding in that the side effects of many currently employed anti-retrovirals are due to inhibition of host cellular DNA polymerases. This means that Green Tea polyphenols inhibit viral replication at low concentrations, low enough to avoid destroying normal cells, which suggests that side-effects from EGCG would be minimal.

As can be seen, Green Tea possesses unique and broad effects. While much research must yet be done to see if all these conclusions will apply to humans, we can safely assume that the wisdom of the ages is not to be ignored. In the future, having a cup of tea might mean more than just enjoying a pleasant beverage.

LEMONGRASS

Scientific Name: *Cymbopogon citratus*
Parts Used: Oil

Recent Scientific Findings

Lemongrass's essential oil contains the monoterpene myrcene, an analgesic, thus confirming Lemongrass tea's traditional use as a mild sedative. One team of researchers concluded that "Terpenes such as myrcene may constitute a lead for the development of new peripheral analgesics with a profile of action different from that of the aspirin-like drugs."

Myrcene was also found to reduce the toxic and mutagenic effect of cyclophosphamide in in vitro experiments. In other words, myrcene may possess antimutagenic properties.

Lemongrass oil has also been reported to possess strong antibacterial activity in vitro against several human pathogens. For instance, a 1988 study found an appreciable increase in activity against *Escherichia coli* and *Staphylococcus aureus*.

Lemongrass oil is also rich in geraniol and citral, both of which may contribute to lowering serum cholesterol levels. In one study involving 22 hypercholesterolemic patients, cholesterol levels were lowered. However, to date there is no laboratory evidence to support Lemongrass' reputed folkloric ability to relieve anxiety.

LETTUCE, WILD

Scientific Name: *Lactuca elongata*
Parts Used: Latex
Dosage: Latex: When used for its sedative effects, the latex of Wild Lettuce was taken in a dose of 3.0 to 12 grams every 24 hours.

Recent Scientific Findings

Lactucarium, found in this and other species of Lettuce, is obtained by wounding the plants in the flowering season when their vessels are filled with juice and so irritable that they often spontaneously burst or are ruptured by very slight accidental injuries.

This fresh milky latex contains a sedative principle known as lactupicrin. The best way to collect this juice is by placing successive small pieces of cotton on the cut stem and throwing them into a little water. After a quantity has accumulated, the water holding in solution the contents of the pieces of cotton is evaporated, and an extract thus procured. An easier way to collect the latex is by macerating the stems and leaves in water, just after the seeds have matured and before the plant decays. The maceration is to be continued for 24 hours, then the liquid is boiled for 2 hours, and finally evaporated in shallow basins.

Lactucarium has very mild pain allaying and calmative effects, somewhat like a weak dose of opium. It may best be employed as a mild sedative. It was also used as a draught in constipation, intestinal disorders such as engorements, and for other gastric upsets.

LICORICE

Scientific Name: *Glycyrrhiza glabra*
Parts Used: Root
Dosage: Root: 1 teaspoon of the root or subterranean stem, boiled in a covered container with 1 1/2 pints of water for about 1/2 hour, at a slow boil. Allow liquid to cool slowly in the *closed* container. Drink cold, 1 swallow or 1 tablespoon at a time, 1 to 2 cups per day.

Recent Scientific Findings

The multitude of pharmacological effects of Licorice rhizomes and roots are practically all attributed to the presence of a triterpene saponin called *glycyrrhizin,* which is about fifty times sweeter than sugar, and has a powerful cortisone-like effect. Several cases have been reported in medical literature in which humans ingesting 6-8 ounces (a very large amount) of licorice candy daily for a period of several weeks are "poisoned" due to the cortisone-like effects of licorice extract in the candy. Proper treatment restores patients to normal. The above amount of this compound is very large compared with the relatively small amount found in supplements.

In addition, Licorice rhizomes and roots have a high mucilage content. When mixed with water, the resulting preparation has a very pleasant odor and taste, and acts as an effective demulcent on irritated mucous membranes, such as accompany a sore throat. One study found that glycyrrhizin was as effective a cough suppressant as codeine. A 1991 experiment with mice found that glycyrrhizin protected against skin cancer. The authors speculated that it might prove useful in protecting against some forms of human cancer as well.

It is not surprising that Licorice and glycyrrhizin have such wide applications. It should be noted that this chemical constitutes only 7 to 10% of the total root (on a dry weight basis). Glycyrrhetic acid (G.A.) is obtained when acid hydrolysis is applied to the main component of licorice. This compound is extensively used in Europe for its anti-inflammatory properties, especially in Addison's disease and peptic ulcer. Some European researchers concluded that G.A. may be preferred to cortisone because it is safer, especially when prolonged treatment is required.

A recent study (1990) demonstrated that G.A. exerts its activity *not* as a *direct effect* but by reducing the conversion of cortisol to cortisone, its biologically inactive product. The authors concluded that hydrocortisone, a "weak anti-inflammatory agent," can be greatly potentiated (i.e., made more powerful) by the addition of 2% GA. To lessen the toxic effects of corticosteroids, the authors suggested that patients use hydrocortisone *together* with GA. Here is another example of the growing marriage between prescription pharmaceuticals and herbal preparations.

Glycyrrhizin has also exhibited anti-viral activity. A 1979 study demonstrated that glycyrrhizin inhibited Epstein-Barr Virus (EBV), cytomegalovirus (CMV), and hepatitis B virus. In Japan, glycyrrhizin has long been successfully used to treat chronic hepatitis B. This has led to speculation that glycyrrhizin holds promise in the treatment of HIV.

A note of caution: Side effects from the ingestion of large amounts of Licorice have been reported. Glycyrrhizin in very large amounts can promote hypokalemia and hypertension. For these reasons people with heart problems and high blood pressure are advised to avoid consuming large quantities of Licorice or its components.

MILK THISTLE

Scientific Name: *Silybum marianum*
Parts Used: Seeds
Dosage: Seeds: 1 teaspoon seeds steeped in 1/2 cup water; 1 to 1 1/2 cupfuls per day, 1 tablespoon or mouthful at a time.

Recent Scientific Findings

One active component extracted from milk thistle seeds, silymarin, is a flavonoid long recognized for its ability to benefit people with liver disorders and as a protective compound against liver-damaging agents as diverse as mushroom toxins, carbon tetrachloride, and other chemicals. This flavonoid demonstrates good antioxidant properties, both *in vivo* and *in vitro*.

Chilean scientists found that silymarin also increases the content of liver glutathione (GSH), an effect *not* known with other closely related flavonoids such as (+)-cyanidanol-3 (cathequin). These experiments also showed an increase of glutathione content and antioxidant activity in the intestine and stomach. The effects selectively occur only in the digestive tract, and not in the kidney, lung, and spleen.

A double blind, prospective, randomized study performed on 170 patients with cirrhosis of the liver supported the fact that silymarin protects the liver. All patients received the same treatment with a mean observation period of 41 months. The 4-year survival rate was significantly higher in silymarin-treated patients than those in the placebo group. No side effects of drug treatment were observed.

Another study found that Milk Thistle may offer us some protection against the toxic side-effects of the common pain-relieving drug acetaminophen, which is a widely used analgesic and fever medication. In overdosage severe hepatotoxicity may result, characterized by glutathione (GSH) depletion, suppression of GSH biosynthesis, and liver damage. GSH is considered the most important biomolecule against chemically-induced cytotoxicity.

Silybin, a soluble form of silymarin, is thought to exert a membrane-stabilizing action which inhibits or prevents lipid peroxidation. Silybin and silymarin may be useful in protecting the liver in many cases besides acetaminophen overdosage. Alcohol also depletes GSH and these flavonoids offer protection for those who continue to drink. Interestingly, silybin dihemisuccinate remains medicine's most important antidote to poisoning by the mushroom toxins a-amantin and phalloidin.

MUSTARD

Scientific Name: *Sinapis alba, S. nigra*
Parts Used: Seeds
Dosage: *Caution:* Mustard plasters can rarely be taken for more than 10 or 15 minutes. As an emetic (especially used in narcotic poisoning), mustard powder was given in the quantity of 3.9-7.7 grams.

Recent Scientific Findings

Black and White Mustard seeds both contain highly irritating so-called "mustard-oil" glycosides, typified by "mustard oil," or allyl isothiocyanate. The irritant effect is mild in water extracts, but in concentrated extracts, the irritation can actually induce blistering. A combination of mild irritation due to the mustard-oil glycosides, in addition to a high fat content, causes the laxative effect of

Mustard seeds. In larger doses, the irritant action of the mustard-oil glycosides causes emesis.

Mustard plasters are still widely used, and their effective utility requires special handling. The mustard plaster is simply a thin layer of deflated Mustard seeds, applied to a piece of paper with a suitable glue. Prior to use, the mustard plaster is dipped into lukewarm (never hot) water. This contact with water sets off a chemical reaction in which the end-product is "mustard oil." The plaster is then applied for a short period of time. While the plaster is in contact with the skin, the blood rushes to the area of application. The additional blood supply serves to produce an anti-inflammatory response, relax muscles, and in general provide relief from muscle strains and similar ailments.

It must be pointed out that the mustard plaster should not be allowed to remain in contact with the skin for any prolonged period of time, or it will result in the formation of blisters. The blisters are very painful and there is always a possibility that infection will result. However, mustard plasters, applied externally for periods up to 15 minutes, will usually not result in blistering, and are quite safe and effective for those whose skin is of normal sensitivity.

Mustard oil itself is used in many proprietary ointments intended for external application for the relief of minor aches and pains, much the same as mustard plaster.

PAPAYA

Scientific Name: *Carica papaya*
Parts Used: Leaf and latex
Dosage: Leaves: The leaves are wrapped directly on wounds. Latex: Latex used as needed; avoid internal use due to presence of protein-digesting properties.

Recent Scientific Findings

The dried latex of the Papaya is marketed under the names papayotin, papain or papoid, and is given to treat dyspepsia and gastric catarrh. In powder form it is applied to treat skin diseases, including warts and tubercle swellings. Much of this medicinal product is supplied from Ceylon and the West Indies. It is still employed as a meat tenderizer and is contained as an additive in one brand of beer to dissolve excess proteins, thereby making the beer more clear.

The enzyme chymopapain, a derivative of the latex of the Papaya, has been used on an experimental basis by neurosurgeons to dissolve herniated ("slipped") intervertebral discs in patients complaining of back pain.

Preliminary research has also revealed cardiac depressant activity when given orally to human adults and cardiotonic activity.

PARSLEY

Scientific Name: *Petroselinum sativum*
Parts Used: Leaf, root, and seeds
Dosage: Leaves: Approximately 1 ounce of leaves to 1 pint of water. Boil water separately and pour over the plant material and steep for 5 to 20 minutes, depending on the desired effect. Drink hot or warm, 1 to 2 cups per day, at bedtime and upon awakening.

Recent Scientific Findings

A great deal of research has been conducted on Parsley's effect on cells and DNA. Some of the medical implications involve the enzymes that are integral to disease resistance response. In vitro studies have shown Parsley has antibacterial and antifungal effects. Unfortunately, little research has occurred to confirm or deny Parsley's folkloric claims as a remedy for liver ailments.

One of Parsley's chemical constituents, Apiol, is a uterine stimulant, as to a lesser extent is another constituent, myristicin. The Russian product "Supetin," comprised of 85% parsley juice, is used to stimulate uterine contractions during labor. At one time, Apiol was used in capsules as an abortifacient. Apiol and myristicin also contribute to Parsley's effectiveness as a diuretic.

Parsley is rich in nutrients, including vitamins A, B, C, and K as well as protein and potassium.

Caution: Use of Parsley should be avoided during pregnancy.

PEPPERMINT

Scientific Name: *Mentha piperita*
Parts Used: Leaves and flowering tops
Dosage: Leaves: Approximately 1/2 ounce of leaves to 1 pint of boiling water. Boil water separately and pour over the plant material and steep for 5-20 minutes, depending on the desired effect. Drink hot or warm, 1 to 2 cups or more per day.

Recent Scientific Findings

Peppermint tea is one of the most common herbal remedies, used primarily as a carminative and intestinal antispasmodic. These effects are all explained on the basis of animal experiments using the essential oil from Peppermint, or purified essential oil constituents, the results of which mimic the effects claimed in humans. This essential oil has a high menthol content. Menthol both stimulates the flow of bile to the stomach and is an antispasmodic.

POMEGRANATE

Scientific Name: *Punica granatum*
Parts Used: Bark, rind, and fruit
Dosage: Root bark: 1 teaspoonful of root bark, chopped small, to 1½ pints of boiling water; slow boil in a covered container for about ½ hour. Allow liquid to cool slowly in the *closed* container. Drink cold, 1 mouthful at a time, over the day, to a maximum of 1 cup total.

Recent Scientific Findings

Of all types of intestinal worm infestations, Pomegranate root bark is most useful in cases of tapeworm. The active principle, discovered in 1878, is the liquid alkaloid pelletierine, which was used in human medicine for a number of years, and then became relegated to veterinary use. Thus, it is well established that root bark preparations of Pomegranate would be effective when used to expel worms from the intestinal tract.

Anyone who has bitten into the peel of a Pomegranate fruit can testify to the highly astringent nature of this material. In fact, it is known that the fruit peel contains about 30 percent of tannin, which is the active astringent substance.

RASPBERRY, RED

Scientific Name: *Rubus spp.*
Parts Used: Leaf
Dosage: Leaves: One teaspoon of the leaf is used per cup of boiling water. Drink cold, 1 to 2 cups per day. During pregnancy: steep ½ ounce with 1 pint of boiling water 3-5 minutes, drink warm, 1 pint per day.

Root bark: The root bark is used in the proportion of one teaspoonful of chopped root bark per 1½ pints of water; boil down to 1 pint, and administer 1 to 2 ounces cold, 3 or 4 times per day.

Recent Scientific Findings

Red Raspberry leaves contain high concentrations of tannins, which is most likely responsible for the antinauseant, antivomiting, antidiarrheal, and astringent effects of this plant. A vast literature exists supporting the numerous folkloric claims for this interesting plant genus. Various species of Raspberry have been shown to: induce ovulation, relax the uterus, act as a diuretic, stimulate immunity, kill viruses (including herpes), control glucose-induced high blood sugar, promote insulin production, kill fungi, and stimulate interferon induction.

Red Raspberry leaf or root tea is an excellent astringent remedy for diarrhea, and will also allay nausea and vomiting. The leaf tea is also drunk during pregnancy to facilitate childbirth, and, as indicated above, will help with "morning sickness."

As the scientific evidence indicates, many species of Raspberry are "super-useful" for a myriad of women's problems. One study showed that Raspberry leaf prevented the typical hyper-growth effects of chronic gonadotrophin on ovaries and uterus, while another study demonstrated that Raspberry leaf relaxes uterine muscles. In the latter study tea concentrates were tested on several species of animal. If the smooth muscle of the uterus was "in tone," the water extract of Raspberry leaf relaxed it. If the muscle was relaxed, the herb caused contractions.

Other studies have found antiviral activity in cell culture against vaccinia virus and strong antiviral activity (in cell culture) against herpes virus II; also antiviral activity has been found against soxsackie virus, influenza virus, polio virus I, and reovirus I.

REISHI MUSHROOM

Scientific Name: *Ganoderma lucidum, G. japonicum*
Parts Used: Cap and stem
Dosage: 2 to 3 grams, in capsule or tablet form, once per day.

Recent Scientific Findings

Long regarded with suspicion by Americans, the mushrooms are now receiving renewed attention owing to the health promoting compounds found in several species. While most of the results reported thus far are based on animal studies, the historical reverence assigned reishi mushrooms by the Japanese tends to support the contention that human studies will produce equally exciting results.

Reishi mushrooms are commercially available in several varieties. *G. lucidum*, the red variety, is the type preferred in Japan. *G. japonicum*, which is darker and softer as well as cultured varieties are also sold. Chinese herb doctors tend not to distinguish these species, using them all, however, only *G. lucidum* has been the subject of intensive research.

A recent study from Korea showed that *Ganoderma* elicited immunopotentiation in mice. Antitumor activity in mice of polysaccharide fractions of these mushrooms was reported from Japan, while Chinese scientists described adaptogenic activity, again in mice. According to this Chinese study a hot water extract was found to enhance a self-protecting mechanism of the central nervous system, improve heart function and correct parasympathetic nerve function. Perhaps most interestingly this study also demonstrated an anti-radiation effect from a polysaccharide fraction.

The immune-enhancing effects ascribed to Reishi mushrooms by the Korean scientists noted above were described as enhancing macrophages and polymorphonuclear leucocytes (two types of fighting cells). Many studies have reported potent antiallergic activity, including antihistamine actions. And, it is now well-established that mushrooms such as Reishi can significantly reduce serum cholesterol and "thin" the blood in a manner similar to aspirin by reducing agglutination of platelets.

A 1990 study involved 15 healthy volunteers and 33 patients with atherosclerotic diseases. When a watery soluble extract was added to the platelets in vitro, the healthy volunteers showed platelet inhibition in relation to dosage.

From the above documentation it appears that the claims of healing properties in these (and other) mushrooms are based on fact not myth. Fears of toxicity should be allayed by the finding that reishi has an LD50 of greater than 5,000 mg/K, with no toxic effect at this high level of consumption even after 30 days of consumption. No toxic effects in humans are to be expected even if a person were to eat 350 grams a day, between 40-300 times the therapeutic dose.

ROSEMARY

Scientific Name: Rosmarinus officinalis
Parts Used: Leaf and flowers
Dosage: 0.5 to 1.0 grams per day of the ground leaf on food, or in capsule or tablet form taken orally.

Recent Scientific Findings

Rosemary's volatile oil is used in rubefacients and carminatives. It is official in the U.S. Pharmacopoeia. A recent study suggested that a Rosemary extract may be a chemopreventive agent for breast cancer. A dietary supplement of the extract "resulted in a significant (47%) decrease in mammary tumor incidence compared to controls."

SAGE

Scientific Name: *Salvia officinalis*
Parts Used: Leaves and flowering tops
Dosage: Leaves: Steep 1 teaspoon leaves in ½ cup water for 30 minutes; take 1 cup per day, 1 tablespoon at a time.

Recent Scientific Findings

The "minor" tranquilizers such as Valium® and Librium®, classified as benzodiazepines, have been widely prescribed since 1960 to treat epilepsy, muscle spasms, sleep problems, and anxiety. They are very effective but quite addictive, with physical dependence demonstrated in humans who have used these agents repeatedly.

If only humankind could have that "perfect" anti-anxiety agent! It would calm without sedating, be non-addictive, and not induce strong muscle relaxation. Does this sound like SOMA, the mythic perfect drug sought for ages?

According to a team of Japanese scientists, the common Chinese variety of Sage may contain the perfect tranquilizing compound within its roots. A single compound found in this plant may become the source of a new tranquilizing agent, acting like Valium without the troublesome side-effects noted above.

The Benzodiazepines act at pharmacologically specific sites in the central nervous system, the central B_2 receptors, to inhibit nerve transmission by enhancing the neurotransmission of GABA (an inhibitor of neurotransmission). The plant-derived compounds described in the above study also interact with the central B_2 receptors. Determined to be diterpene quinones, so-called tanshinones, they chemically differ from all the other known natural and synthetic B_2 receptors yet discovered.

The most potent of these tanshinones is Miltirone. In experiments with mice it was found to diminish anxiety *without* producing sedation or muscle relaxation, and without diminishing performance or producing addiction.

Other studies have found Sage to be of some use in soothing and regulating menopausal problems, possessing antibacterial activity in vitro against several human pathogens, and exhibiting anti-yeast activity in vitro against Candida albicans and antiviral activity in cell culture against herpes simplex virus II, influenza virus A2, vaccinia virus, and polio virus II.

SARSAPARILLA

Scientific Name: *Smilaxaristolochiaefolia, S. medica, S. officinalis*
Parts Used: Root
Dosage: Root: Boil 1 teaspoon of the root in a covered container of 1 1/2 pints of water for about 1/2 hour, at a slow boil. Allow liquid to cool slowly in the closed container. Drink cold, 1 swallow or 1 tablespoon at a time, 1 to 2 cups per day.

Recent Scientific Findings

Commonly regarded as tonic, diaphoretic, and diuretic, Sarsaparilla in actuality is probably no more than a mild gastric irritant due to its saponin content.

Sarsasapogenin and smilagenin are steroidal aglycones with potential use as precusors for the synthetic production of cortisone and other steroidal drugs. The plant possesses diuretic action, stimulating the excretion of uric acid. Sarsaparilla root extracts have been observed to have anti-tubercle bacillus activity in culture studies.

SASSAFRAS

Scientific Name: *Sassafras albidium*
Parts Used: Root bark
Dosage: Root bark: For those who may wish to defy the official ban, it is interesting to note that in former times this plant was very frequently used as a spring tonic. One cup of boiling water was added to a teaspoonful of the granulated

root bark. It was taken cold, a mouthful at a time, to a maximum of 1 cup daily. useful externally for poison ivy and poison oak.

Recent Scientific Findings

The aromatic oil is still utilized as an antiseptic and as a flavoring agent. The essential oil from the root bark of Sassafras has been experimentally determined to have antiseptic properties, and if applied externally would undoubtedly have such an effect, as reported in folkloric use.

Water extracts of Sassafras root bark continue to be used widely, especially in North America, as refreshing aromatic teas. Such teas contain small amounts (about 7-10 milligrams per cup) of a chemical compound known as safrole. In the early 1960s it was found that safrole, when fed to rodents in their diet, resulted in liver damage, and more specifically, liver cancer, in a high percentage of animals. This caused the U.S. Food and Drug Administration to prohibit the sale of safrole-containing materials, such as Sassafras root bark, for use in foods and flavors. However, despite an official ban, Sassafras root and root bark remain as an item of commerce in the United States, and are still widely used.

Of importance is that safrole itself does not produce cancer in animals. It must be converted by the animal to a substance containing one additional hydroxy group, i.e., 1-hydroxysafrole. The latter substance is termed a proximate carcinogen. 1-hydroxysafrole is produced by several animal species, including rats, mice, and digs, when safrole is administered orally.

Interestingly enough, in 1977 the results of a study conducted in Switzerland was published in which safrole was taken orally by one human adult, and the proximate carcinogen 1-hydorxysafrole could be found in the urine of this individual. It is well known that chemical compounds may be converted differently by different species. If additional confirming experiments are carried out in humans, and it is found that safrole is not changed to a carcinogen, the official ban on the sale of Sassafras root bark may be removed.

SEAWEEDS

Scientific Name: *Geldium, Gracilaria,* and *Pterocladia* spp. (Agar-Agar); *Lyngbya lagerheimii* and *Phormidium tenue* (Blue-Green Algae), *Laminaria* spp. (Brown Algae, Kelp), *Chlorella* spp. (Chlorella), *Chondrus crispus* (Irish Moss)
Parts Used: Whole plant
Dosage: Agar: It should be eaten daily as a cereal in the amount of 7 to 15 grams. Other Species: Follow the label directions of commercial preparations.
Dextran sulfate should be taken under medical supervision.

Recent Scientific Findings

An entire book has been written that is devoted to "marine algae in pharmaceutical science." Marine flora are shown to possess numerous medicinal properties, including antibiotic, antiviral, antimicrobial in general, and antifungal.

Japanese food is in vogue in Western nations, primarily because of the low fat, low calorie, high-fiber aspects. Wakame (a brown kelp, Undaria), Kombu (Laminaria), and Nori (Porphyra) which is used to wrap around rice for sushi, all contain active antitumor compounds.

These sea vegetables protect us against cancers of the digestive tract due to at least four known factors:

1. The alginic acid content swells in the intestine thus diluting potential carcinogens.

2. Some contain beta-sitosterol, a potent anti-cancer compound.

3. They may contain antibiotic compounds which inhibit the growth of several different gram-positive and gram-negative bacteria known to potentiate carcinogens in the colon.

4. They may possess antioxidant activity.

Agar-Agar

This sea plant has a very high concentration of polysaccharide mucilage, which swells and is very slimy when moistened. This mucilage is responsible for the laxative effect of agar, exerting a type of lubricant effect.

When used as a laxative, Agar should be taken with large amounts of water, and never dry. It usually will not produce a laxative effect with a single dose, but must be used regularly. Its function is very similar to that of vegetable cellulose foods and of bran. As a good bulk laxative, it may also be added to cereals, soups, cakes, or any other food without altering its effect. If the constipation is stubborn, Cascara (see Cascara Sagrada) bark is added to precipitate action.

Blue-Green Algae

Most of the recent attention to the Seaweeds has centered around dextran sulfate's possible action against the AIDS virus. Dextran sulfate is created when dextran is boiled with chlorosulfonic acid. It is a sulfate ester not a sulfonic acid. Dextran sulfate has been used for more than 30 years in Japan, primarily as an intravenous drug that reduces clotting and lowers blood cholesterol. Dextran sulfate also inactivates the herpes simplex virus.

In a 1987 letter to The Lancet, two Japanese researchers reported that dextran sulfate blocked the binding of HIV-1 to T-lymphocytes as well as blocking the transfer of HIV from cell to cell by cell fusion. The authors followed this with another paper that maintained that dextran sulfate could work synergistically with AZT in vitro.

Recently, Dr. K. R. Gustafson and other scientists at the National Cancer Institute (U.S.) reported that cellular extracts from cultured Blue-Green Algae protected human T cells from infection with the AIDS virus. In test-tube experiments pure compounds extracted from these algae also proved to be "strikingly active against HIV-1."

These algae were originally collected in Hawaii and the Palau Islands (Micronesia) and then cultured. The original technique for culturing such marine organisms and producing an extract (which later proved to be cytotoxic) was pioneered by my first professor of pharmacology, Dr. T.R. Norton. It was in 1968 in Dr. Norton's basement laboratory at Leahi Hospital of the University of Hawaii School of Medicine where I was first introduced to the search for medicines from plants.

The AIDS virus killing compounds just discovered in the Blue-Green Algae are classified as sulfolipids. These lipids are found within the structures of chloroplast membranes and occur widely in other algae, higher plants and microorganisms which conduct photosynthesis.

Initial clinical trials with dextran sulfate treatment for HIV indicate a fairly frequent improvement of general well-being. Consistent changes in T-cell counts were not noted. A John Hopkins University study confirmed the initial results from a study at San Francisco General Hospital that dextran sulfate is poorly absorbed when given orally.

Brown Algae

I first learned of the anti-cancer and antithrombotic effects of the brown algae from a Japanese colleague. True, I had long believed that mankind would once again "return to the sea," by adding the aquatic plants to his armamentarium of terrestrial medicinals. But my attention was not galvanized until I learned about fucoidan.

Recent research has shown that the main active component with antitumor activity in edible seaweeds is likely a type of sulphated polysaccharide, fucoidan. The same compound has been shown to be responsible for anticoagulant and fibrinolytic activities in animal studies. Another researcher, utilizing epidemiological and biological data, speculates that the brown kelp seaweed *Laminaria* is "an important factor contributing to the relatively low breast cancer rates reported in Japan."

Brown algae also contains dextran sulfate. See the above discussion under Blue-Green Algae for further information.

Chlorella

These microscopic species of algae possess distinct biological activities and are certain to take their place among the better-known marine organisms. All that has been said about the other species of seaweed is also applicable to the various unicellular marine algae, especially species of *Chlorella*.

Numerous animal studies have demonstrated antitumor activity, antiviral activity, and interferon inducing effects. The antitumor activity was observed specifically against mammary tumors, against leukemia, ascitic sarcoma, and liver cancer. A glycolipid fraction was tested which showed immune-enhancing effects in mice, most likely it was chlorellin.

An extract of Chlorella was found to have antiviral activity against cytomegalovirus (in mice) and against equine encephalitis virus (horse).

Immune stimulation by extract of Chlorella was observed due to induction of interferon production in mice infected with estomegalovirus (murine) and enhanced natural killer cell production was observed in mice infested with estomegalovirus as well as in mice with lymphoma-YAC-I.

Antihypertensive and antihyperlipedimic activity were observed with the protein fraction derived from Chlorella.

Irish Moss

Irish Moss is commonly used as a stabilizer in various foods, especially dairy products.

Experimental results have shown that Irish Moss may reduce high blood pressure. A product has been patented containing an extract of Irish Moss. The manufacturers claim the extract treats ulcers.

Other promising areas that have been observed in preliminary testing and warrant further investigation include Irish Moss' properties as a demulcent, an anti-inflammatory, an immune-stimulant, antibacterial activity against Streptococcus mutans, and lymphocyte blastogenesis stimulant activity.

SHIITAKE MUSHROOM

Scientific Name: *Lentinus edodes*
Parts Used: Cap and stem
Dosage: Whole Plant: Approximately 1 ounce of the chopped mushroom to 1 pint of water. Boil water separately and pour over the mushroom and steep for 5 to 20 minutes, depending on the desired effect. Drink hot or warm, 1 to 2 cups per day.

Recent Scientific Findings

When I first studied medical mycology, over 20 years ago, Wilson and Plunkett's classic text provoked such fear and revulsion through the color photos of rare fungous diseases of man that I vowed to never eat another mushroom! All fungi became a source of dread for me.

Within the past few years I have since changed my view of these "lower" plants. The mushrooms are not only acceptable to me but have become highly coveted, owing to their documented immuno-stimulant, cholesterol-lowering, and antitumor activities.

Extracts of Shiitake have been shown to inhibit a number of different cancerous tumors in animal experiments. A principle antitumor compound isolated from this species *lentinan* does not appear to kill tumor cells directly but inhibits tumor growth by stimulating immune-function.

Lentinan appears to function by activating macrophages which then engulf cancerous cells. This activation is again via an indirect route—T-helper cells are stimulated which increase the effectiveness of macrophages.

The AIDS epidemic has fostered interest in any helpful compounds and lentinan is now a high priority item. A highly publicized letter to the prestigious medical journal *The Lancet* (October 20, 1984) was signed by Robert Gallo, one of the co-discoverer of the HIV Virus, and two French researchers from the Pasteur Institute. In it the authors concluded that lentinan "may prove to be effective in AIDS or pre-AIDS or for HIV carriers." After intravenous administration of lentinan with two Japanese patients, HTLV-I and HTLV-III antibodies disappeared.

The use of lentinan to treat AIDS is still in its early stages. In Japan, a few hemophiliacs infected with HIV have been administered lentinan. After several months treatment, there was a modest boost in T4 cells while macrophages and NK cells showed increased activity.

Unfortunately, despite repeated requests to subject this drug to human trials, based on its long history of usage for cancer treatment in Japan, nothing much has been done by governmental authorities in the U.S.

This is odd considering the long list of studies showing lentinan's antiviral properties; interferon inducing, natural killer cell enhancing, phagocytosis rate enhancing, as well as numerous antitumor studies. The *in vitro* inhibition of HIV by an extract of this mushroom is not, of itself, highly significant owing to the many substances known to kill this virus. However, taken together with all of the above evidence, it is safe to assume that Shiitake is all that it is claimed to be.

Caution: Skin and respiratory allergic reactions have been observed in workers involved in the commercial production of Shiitake.

SPEARMINT

Scientific Name: *Mentha spicata*
Parts Used: Leaves and flowering tops
Dosage: Leaves and Flowering tops: Approximately ½ ounce of leaves and flowering tops to 1 pint of water. Boil water separately and pour over the plant material and steep for 5 to 20 minutes, depending on the desired effect. Drink hot or warm, 1 to 2 cups or more per day.

Recent Scientific Findings

The leaves and flowering tops of Spearmint owe their pleasant and aromatic properties, as well as characteristic taste, to a volatile oil. The major active principle in the oil is a simple terpene derivative, carvone. Refer to Peppermint, for further information. This plant is the same in action, only weaker due to the fact it does not contain menthol. Its use is largely a matter of taste preference.

THYME

Scientific Name: *Thymus vulgaris*
Parts Used: Herb
Dosage: Herb: Approximately 1/2 ounce of herb to 1 pint of water. Boil water separately and pour over the plant material and steep for 50 to 20 minutes, depending on the desired effect. Drink hot or warm, 1 to 2 cups per day, at bedtime and upon awakening.

Recent Scientific Findings

The active principle, a simple terpene, thymol or thymic acid, has been shown to have disinfectant properties equal to those of carbolic acid. Thymol has been shown to have antiseptic value, expectorant and bronchodilator effects in animal as well as human experiments. Thymol additionally releases entrapped gas in the stomach and relaxes the smooth muscle of that organ. This explains the use of Thyme to alleviate the symptoms of colic and flatulence.

Externally, thymol and thymol- containing plants act as rubefacients. That is, thymol causes an increased blood flow to the area of application, which then results in relief of inflammation and pain.

TURMERIC

Scientific Name: *Curcuma longa*
Parts Used: Rhizome
Dosage: 1 to 2 grams per day in food or take capsules/tablets.

Recent Scientific Findings

Currently, Turmeric is used in India to treat anorexia, liver disorders, cough, diabetic wounds, rheumatism, and sinusitis. In one study Turmeric extract was tested for its anticarcinogenic and antimutagenic properties. Laboratory (non-human) experiments it was found that this ancient spice reduced both the number of tumors in mice and the mutagenicity of benzo(a)pyrene (BP) and two other potent mutagens, NPD and DMBA.

Preventing cancer now receives the attention it has long deserved. Numerous biochemical and epidemiological studies have demonstrated diet's role in modulating the development of cancer. Laboratory experiments have established that the active principle of Turmeric (curcumin) is a potent anti-mutagenic agent.

For those interested in *how* curcumin may act to prevent cancer we turn again to the by-now all pervasive theory of free-radical inactivation. The test carcinogens BP and DMBA are metabolically activated to proximate mutagenic/carcinogenic epoxides, which then bind to macromolecules. One study's authors concluded that since curcumin is a potent antioxidant, it may scavenge the epoxides and prevent binding to macromolecules. In other words, this spice's cell-protective properties are similar to nutrient antioxidants, vitamins C and E, which inhibit free radical reactions.

This type of herb is known as a non-steroidal anti-inflammatory (NSAID). Curcumin inhibits cycloxygenase and lipoxygenase enzymes. Curcumin has three main mechanisms of action: 1) antioxidant activity; 2) lipoxygenase inhibitor; and 3) cycloxygenase inhibition. By inhibiting the associated biochemical pathways, inflammation is curtailed. Modern science thus confirms what traditional healers have known for centuries. Namely, that the fresh juice from the rhizome will reduce swelling in recent bruises, wounds and insect bites; and that the dried powdered root kills parasites, relieves head colds and arthritic aches. (Interestingly, this spice has sometimes been used to adulterate ginger.)

A 1991 pharmacological review confirmed many of Turmeric's folkloric effects, including wound healing, gastric mucosa protection, antispasmodic activity, reduction of intestinal gas formation, protection of liver cells, increasing bile production, diminishing platelet aggregation (i.e. blood clumping), lowering serum cholesterol (at very high doses), antibacterial properties, antifungal properties, and potential antitumor activity. While most of the above effects were demonstrated with intravenous extracts in animals, they do parallel folkloric claims in humans and are not to be dismissed as "experimental" or "trivial."

Turmeric's benefits for arthritis treatment have been demonstrated in human clinical trials. A herbal formula of Turmeric, Ashwagandha, and Boswellin was evaluated in a randomized, double-blind, placebo-controlled study. After a one-month evaluation period 12 patients with osteoarthritis were given the herbal formula or placebo for three months. The patients were evaluated every two weeks. After a 15 day wash-out period, the treatment was reversed with the placebo patients receiving the drug and vice versa. Again results were evaluated over a three month period. The patients treated with the herbal formula showed a significant drop in severity of pain and disability score.

WINTERGREEN

Scientific Name: *Gaultheria procumbens*
Parts Used: Leaves and flowering tops
Dosage: Leaves and Flowering tops: One teaspoon of the plant to 1 cup of boiling water, steep for 5 to 20 minutes and drink cold, 1 cup per day, 1 mouthful at a time.

Recent Scientific Findings

Some of the medicinal actions can be explained on the basis of the methyl salicylate contained in the oil, which is closely related to acetylsalicylic acid, or aspirin.

QUERCITIN

(A natural flavone derivative widely distributed in the plant world.)

Quercitin is the commonest flavonoid in higher plants. It is usually present as a glycoside (example: rutin, isoquercitrin, quercitrin, hyperin, and quercimeritrin), but is also isolated in the free state from the families *Compositae, Passiflorae, Rhamnaceae,* and *Solanaceae* (where it mainly occurs on leaf surfaces, in fruits, and in bud extracts).

Quercitin is a powerful antioxidant that decreases the concentration of superoxide anions in enzymic and nonenzymic systems. A recent animal study demonstrated antiulcer and gastroprotective effects, especially against ethanol injury. The cyto-protective activity was effected through several interacting pathways involving stimulation of prostaglandin and inhibition of leukotriene production and through Quercitin's antioxidant properties. Pretreating the experimental animals with 200 mg/kg (a very high dose!) 120 minutes before administering ethanol was found to be the most effective dosage in prevention necrosis.

Commonly Known Antioxidant Plants

Hundreds of plants have been studied and found to possess antioxidant properties. The following list consists of the English names of some plants you probably will recognize.

Some commonly known antioxidant plants include: plantain, leek, onion, garlic, angelica, celery, peanut, bearberry, areca nut, horseradish, tarragon, mugwort, oats, borage, frankincense, tea (black and green), bell peppers (green, red, cayenne, chile, paprika, pimento, etc.), papaya, cinnamon, citrus, coriander, dogwood, cumin, turmeric, lemongrass, Siberian ginseng, eucalyptus, licorice, ivy, elecampane, nettle, bay laurel, lavender, motherwort, hoarhound, balm, mint, pennyroyal, bergamot, mace and nutmeg, myrtle, catnip, basil, olive, marjoram, oregano, rice, ginseng, American ginseng, opium poppy, beans (green, kidney, pinto, etc.), allspice, anise, betel leaf, black pepper, evergreen oak, rosemary, blackberry, raspberry, sage, schizandra, saw palmetto, sesame, spinach, betony, boneset, cloves, cocoa, thyme, cranberry, and ginger.

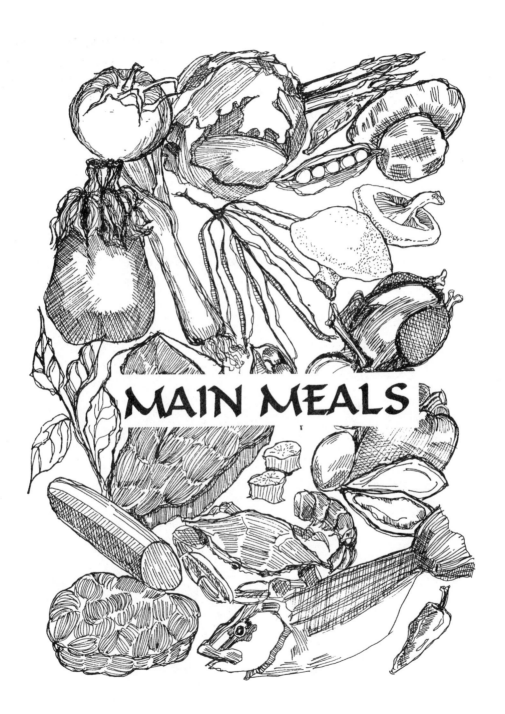

MAIN MEALS

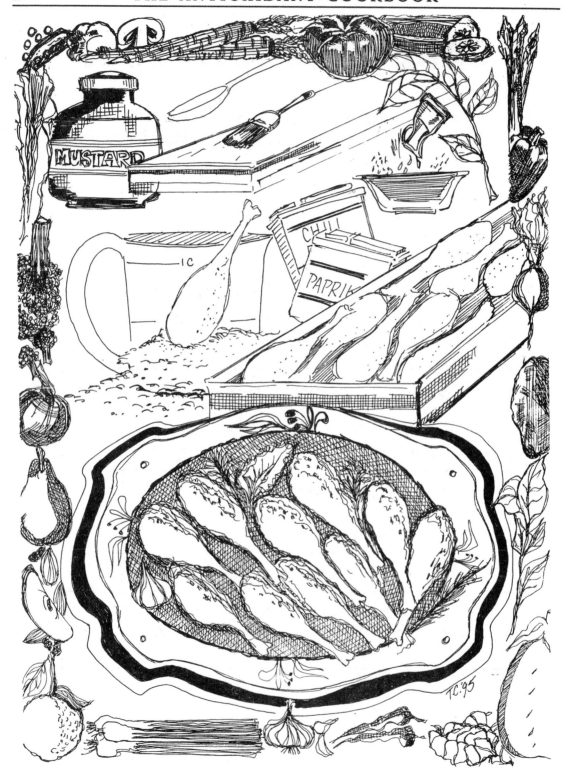

BAKED CHICKEN LEGS

10   chicken drumsticks, skinless
1   teaspoon safflower oil (to brush baking dish with)
1½   teaspoons dry mustard
¾   teaspoon paprika
¼   teaspoon chili flakes
2   teaspoons rice vinegar
1   cup soft bread crumbs

1. Brush baking dish with oil.

2. Mix spice with the vinegar, spread over the chicken pieces.

3. Coat chicken with crumbs. Set pieces in baking dish.

4. Baked covered until tender, approximately 25 minutes.

Rich in the following Antioxidant Nutrients:

Vitamin A	Beta Carotene
Vitamin C	Alpha Carotene
Vitamin E	Lycopene

Plant Antioxidants:

Paprika
Chili Flakes
Safflower Oil
Rice Vinegar

To enhance antioxidant quotient, add the following: After cooking, add to plate: fresh basil leaves sprinkled over baked food.

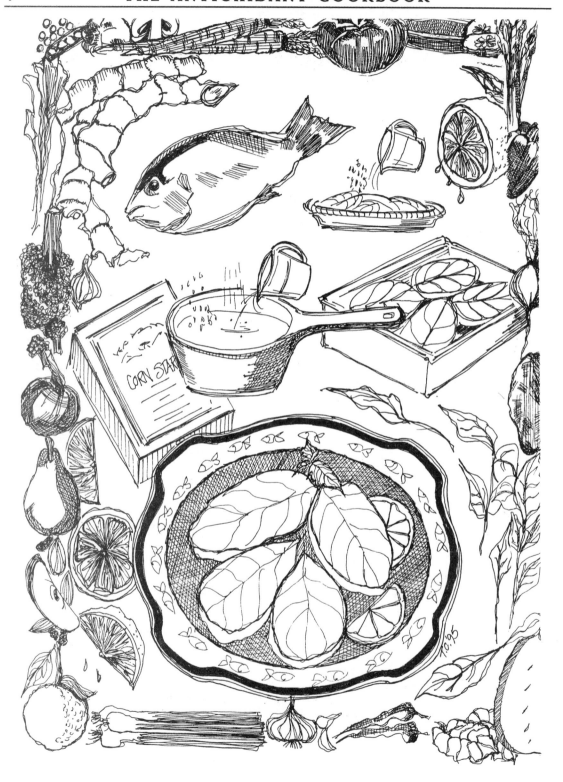

BAKED SNAPPER

4   6 ounce snapper filets
1/2 cup orange juice
1/2 teaspoon minced ginger

1. Combine orange juice and ginger, and marinate fish in this mixture for 30 minutes.

2. Bake, uncovered, at 400 degrees for 20 minutes.

Sauce:

1   can mandarin oranges, drained, reserve the juice (additional orange juice, if needed. You will need 3/4 cup of juice total)
2   teaspoons cornstarch
1/2 teaspoon minced ginger

1. Combine juice and cornstarch in a small saucepan. Bring to a boil, reduce heat, stirring constantly, until mixture has thickened. Remove from heat.

2. Add mandarin orange slices and ginger. Pour over fish and serve immediately.

Rich in the following Antioxidant Nutrients:

Vitamin A	Beta Carotene
Vitamin C	Alpha Carotene
Vitamin E	Lycopene

Plant Antioxidants:
Orange (citrus limonene)
Ginger

To enhance antioxidant quotient, add the following: After cooking, add fresh slices of orange on top of Baked Snapper.

BEEF STIR-SAUTÉED

1	pound flank steak, partially frozen, cut into very thin slices
2	teaspoons cornstarch
1	teaspoons grated fresh ginger
2	teaspoons sesame oil
1	red bell pepper, cut into strips (batonette)
1	papaya, peeled, seeded, cut into large dice
2	tablespoons (brewed) soy sauce, plus 1 tablespoon rice vinegar, combined
1	teaspoon minced garlic

1. Combine soy sauce, vinegar mixture, ginger and cornstarch. Coat meat with this mixture.

2. Heat half of the oil in large sauté or wok. Add garlic and red bell pepper. Sauté for 2 minutes. Set aside.

3. Add remaining oil. Add meat. Stir-fry 1 to 2 minutes, until meat is lightly browned. Add in garlic, red pepper and papaya. Heat through. Serve over steamed white rice.

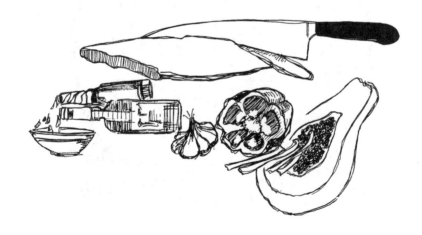

Rich in the following Antioxidant Nutrients:

Vitamin A	Beta Carotene
Vitamin C	Alpha Carotene
Vitamin E	Lycopene

Plant Antioxidants:

Red Bell Pepper
Ginger
Sesame Oil
Papaya
Garlic
Rice Vinegar

To enhance antioxidant quotient, add the following: After cooking, add fresh sliced ginger and papaya to dish, on top.

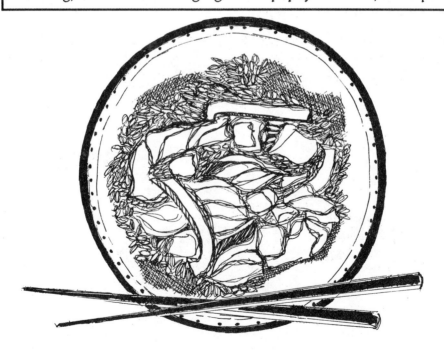

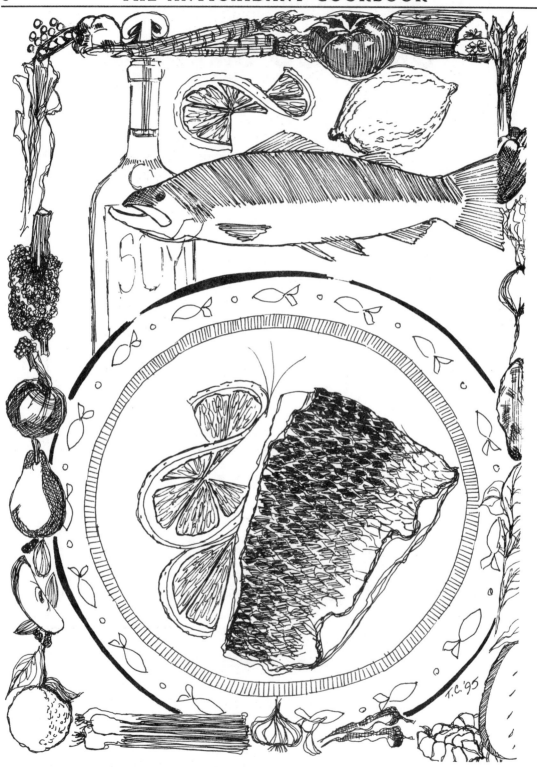

BROILED SALMON

¼   cup (brewed) soy sauce
3   tablespoons lemon juice
½   salmon, cut lengthwise, skinless side up, center bone
    removed (approximately 2 pounds of fish)

1. Combine soy and lemon juices.

2. Baste skinless side of the fish with the mixture.

3. Place under the broiler approximately 15 minutes basting every 3 minutes. Check to insure it does not burn.

* A mixture of the same sauce you used for basting is a nice accompaniment for the cooked fish, with antioxidant-rich spices added to taste.

Rich in the following Antioxidant Nutrients:

Vitamin A	Beta Carotene
Vitamin C	Alpha Carotene
Vitamin E	Lycopene

Plant Antioxidants:

Soy
Lemon (Citrus Limonene)

To enhance antioxidant quotient, add the following: Antioxidant-rich spices (to taste): paprika, garlic, ginger, turmeric. After cooking, add lemon slices to top of broiled salmon.

BURGUNDY BEEF STEW

2	pounds lean ground sirloin
1	teaspoon safflower oil
1	teaspoon garlic chopped
1	medium white onion, finely chopped
1/2	pound mushrooms, sliced
1	cup burgundy wine
2	cups beef broth
6	medium tomatoes, peeled, seeded and chopped
4	medium carrots, peeled and sliced diagonally
1	bay leaf
1/4	teaspoon thyme
2	cups cauliflower florets
2	medium new potatoes, peeled and grated Italian parsley, chopped to garnish

1. In large heavy dutch oven, brown meat in oil.

2. Add onion and garlic to the pan. Cook until onion is slightly brown.

3. Stir in all other ingredients and bring to a boil. Reduce heat and simmer for 20 minutes. Garnish with parsley.

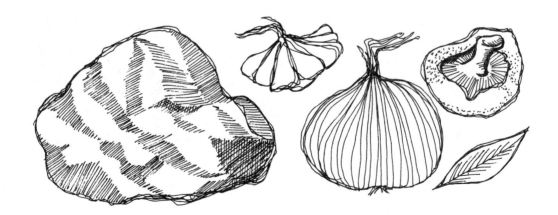

Rich in the following Antioxidant Nutrients:

Vitamin A   Beta Carotene
Vitamin C   Alpha Carotene
Vitamin E   Lycopene

Plant Antioxidants:

Parsley, Italian
Safflower oil
Garlic
Onion
Mushrooms
Burgundy wine
Tomatoes
Carrots
Bay
Thyme

To enhance antioxidant quotient, add the following: After cooking, add fresh chopped parsley, carrots, and onions to top of dish, as a garnish.

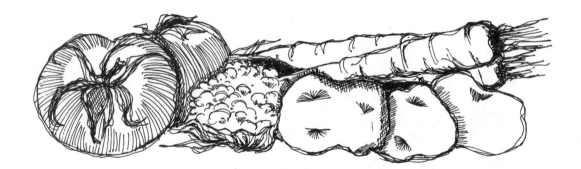

CALAMARI & LINGUINI

12	ounces linguini noodles, cooked al dente
2	tablespoons olive oil
1	pound calamari steaks (4)
1	tablespoon minced garlic
½	cup dry white wine
4	medium tomatoes, peeled and crushed, reserve the liquid
½	cup tomato juice
3	tablespoons Italian parsley, chopped, reserve 1 tablespoon for garnish
½	teaspoon dried oregano
½	teaspoon lemon juice
	salt and pepper to taste

1. Cook linguini noodles, al dente. Drain. Set aside.

2. Pat dry calamari steaks. Rub with lemon juice and season with salt and pepper.

3. In a nonstick sauté pan heat oil. Put calamari steaks in pan and cook approximately 2 minutes on each side. Add garlic to pan. Cook an additional 2 minutes. (If steaks are cooked in 2 batches, divide garlic accordingly.) Set aside.

4. Add wine to sauté pan. Reduce to 3 tablespoons. Stir in tomatoes, tomato juice, parsley and oregano. Simmer over medium heat for approximately 15 minutes, until sauce thickens. Toss with linguini noodles.

5. Place calamari steaks under broiler, to warm, then place them on top of noodles. Garnish with remaining chopped parsley.

Rich in the following Antioxidant Nutrients:

Vitamin A   Beta Carotene
Vitamin C   Alpha Carotene
Vitamin E   Lycopene

Plant Antioxidants:

Olive Oil
Garlic
Tomatoes
Parsley, Italian
Oregano
Lemon (Citrus Bioflavonoids)
Pepper

To enhance antioxidant quotient, add the following: After cooking add sliced red and green fresh bell peppers to dish as a garnish.

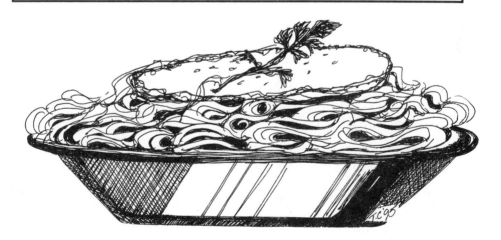

CALIFORNIA PAELLA

2	boneless, skinless chicken breasts
1	pound medium raw mussels
1/2	pound medium raw shrimp (in the shell)
1	pound Italian sausage (turkey)(approximately 4)
3	tablespoons Italian (flatleaf) parsley, chopped
1	cup long grain rice (rinsed until water is clear)
2 1/4	cups hot chicken broth
1	medium white onion, chopped
1	tablespoon garlic, minced
4	medium tomatoes, peeled, seeded and chopped
1	medium red bell pepper, julienne
1	teaspoon dried oregano
1/2	teaspoon paprika
1/4	pound fresh green beans, thinly sliced, 5 ounces frozen peas may be substituted here
2	tablespoons olive oil
	salt and pepper to taste

1. In a large heavy sauté pan/skillet cook sausages. Remove from pan. Allow to cool. Slice the sausage into 1/2" pieces.

2. Add olive oil to sauté pan/skillet, which you have dry washed. Lightly brown, only half cook the chicken pieces. Remove from pan.

3. In remaining fat/oil sauté onion and garlic, until translucent. Remove from heat. Add broth, rice, oregano, paprika, salt and pepper, bring to a boil. Reduce heat. Cover and simmer for 15 minutes.

4. Add tomatoes, parsley, red bell pepper and green beans. Cover and simmer until rice is tender (approximately 5 minutes).

5. Stir in chicken and sausage and arrange seafood over the rice mixture. Cover, and cook for 4 - 6 minutes. (This will steam the mussels open and cook the shrimp.)

Rich in the following Antioxidant Nutrients:

Vitamin A	Beta Carotene
Vitamin C	Alpha Carotene
Vitamin E	Lycopene

Plant Antioxidants:

Parsley, Italian
Onion
Garlic
Tomatoes
Red Bell Pepper
Oregano
Green Beans/Peas
Paprika

To enhance antioxidant quotient, add the following: After cooking, add fresh slices of mango to the top of the paella as a garnish.

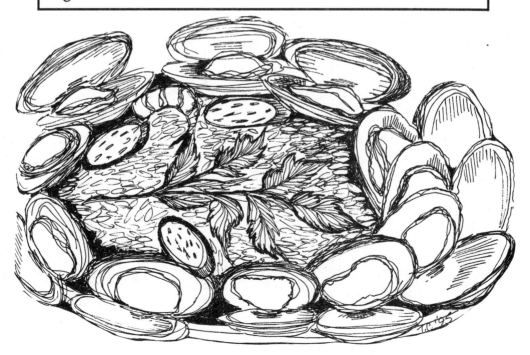

CASSEROLE CHICKEN

(modified to Baked Chicken)

2	medium sized fryers, halved, skinned (approximately 5 pounds total weight)
4	apples (Golden or Red Delicious) cored, peeled and sliced
3	medium carrots (rough cut)
4	shallots (peeled and halved)
1	cup apple juice
1	tablespoon walnut oil
1/2	cup dried cherries
1/2	cup honey mustard
	salt and pepper to season

1. Brush interior of dutch oven, or heavy roasting pan (not glass) with walnut oil. Add the sliced apples, carrots, shallots and cherries, and 1 tablespoon of the apple juice. *Sweat just until they are softened (2 to 3 minutes). Pour remaining apple juice over mixture. Remove from heat.

2. Place chicken pieces on top of sautéed fruits and vegetables. Coat chicken pieces, using basting brush, with honey mustard.

3. Bake in the oven at 375, covered, for approximately 30 minutes. Uncover. Coat chicken with mustard. Cook for 10 additional minutes.

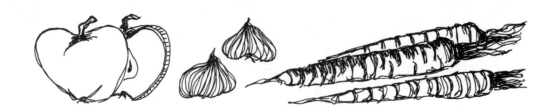

Rich in the following Antioxidant Nutrients:

Vitamin A	Beta Carotene
Vitamin C	Alpha Carotene
Vitamin E	Lycopene

Plant Antioxidants:

Apples
Carrots
Shallots
Walnut oil
Cherries
Pepper

To enhance antioxidant quotient, add the following: After cooking, add toasted sesame seeds, fresh apple slices, and cherries to the top of the chicken.

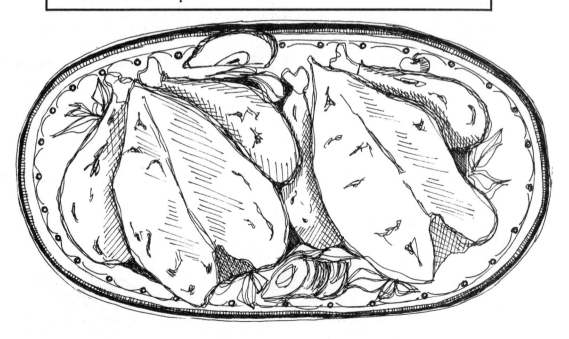

CHICKEN CACCIATORE

1	large frying chicken, skinless, cut up
2	ounces olive oil
1/2	pound mushrooms, sliced
2	tablespoons garlic, minced
1	cup tomato puree
1/2	cup white wine
2	medium white onions, diced
6	roma tomatoes, chopped
1	tablespoon, chopped basil leaves
1/2	teaspoon dry oregano
1	medium zucchini, thinly sliced
1	red bell pepper, julienne

1. Sauté mushrooms in one teaspoon of the olive oil in a non-stick pan.

2. In heavy large skillet put in remaining oil. Brown chicken, on all sides, over medium heat. Remove from pan.

3. To the same skillet add the garlic and onion, cook until onion is translucent.

4. Add puree, wine, basil, zucchini, peppers, bring to a boil.

5. Add chicken and mushrooms. Lower heat and simmer for 25-30 minutes.

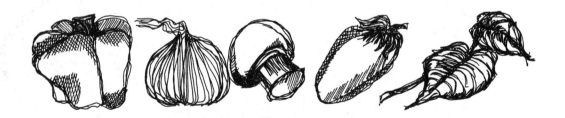

Rich in the following Antioxidant Nutrients:

Vitamin A	Beta Carotene
Vitamin C	Alpha Carotene
Vitamin E	Lycopene

Plant Antioxidants:

Olive Oil
Garlic
Tomatoes
White Wine
Onion
Basil
Oregano
Zucchini
Red Bell Pepper

To enhance antioxidant quotient, add the following: After cooking, add a combination of fresh chopped oregano, fresh chopped basil, and ground black pepper to the top of the cacciatore.

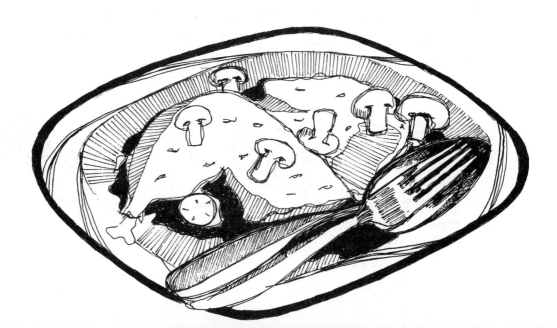

CHICKEN OASIS

1	chicken (fryer cut-up, skinless)
1	medium white onion. coarsely chopped
2	cups chicken broth
2	leeks, white parts only, coarsely chopped
2	large carrots, peeled, julienne
1	celery stalk, chopped
1/4	pound mushrooms, sliced
1	green bell pepper, seeded, cored and chopped
1	tablespoon minced garlic
1/2	cup white wine
6	medium tomatoes, peeled and quartered
1/4	cup raisins
2	teaspoons olive oil
1	teaspoon corn starch
1	teaspoon cumin
1	tablespoon coriander
2	teaspoons paprika
	Salt, pepper and to taste

1. Dust chicken pieces with paprika.

2. In heavy dutch oven heat the olive oil.

3. Brown the chicken then add onions, leeks, celery, green pepper, carrots, and mushrooms. Cook until vegetables are al dente, approximately 2 minutes.

4. Add garlic and cook for an additional minute.

5. Add coriander, cumin, salt and pepper. (Dissolve the cornstarch into 1/4 cup of the broth. Add to the mixture.) Slowly stir in 1 3/4 cups of the broth and wine.

6. Add tomatoes and raisins and simmer for 20 minutes. Serve over cous-cous.

Rich in the following Antioxidant Nutrients:

Vitamin A   Beta Carotene
Vitamin C   Alpha Carotene
Vitamin E   Lycopene

Plant Antioxidants:

Onion
Green Bell Pepper
Leeks
Garlic
Carrots
White Wine
Celery
Tomatoes
Mushrooms
Raisins
Olive Oil
Cumin
Coriander
Paprika
Pepper

To enhance antioxidant quotient, add the following: After cooking, sprinkle fresh chopped celery and cayenne pepper on the top of the dish.

CHICKEN & TURKEY SAUSAGE PAELLA

3	boneless, skinless chicken breasts, cut into strips
6	hot Italian sausages
1	tablespoon olive oil
2	teaspoons minced garlic
1	medium white onion, chopped
1/2	medium green bell pepper, diced
1	medium red bell pepper, julienne
1	teaspoon oregano
1/2	teaspoon paprika
1/4	teaspoon tabasco sauce
1	cup diced tomatoes
1	cup long grain rice (rinsed until water is clear)
2	cups hot chicken broth

1. In a large heavy sauté pan/skillet cook sausages. Remove from pan. Allow to cool. Slice the sausage into 1/2" pieces.

2. Add olive oil to dry washed pan, and lightly brown, only half cook chicken pieces. Remove from pan.

3. In remaining fat/oil sauté garlic, onion, red bell pepper.

4. Add chicken, sausage, rice, broth, oregano, paprika, tabasco, tomatoes to pan and bring to a boil. Reduce heat. Cover and simmer for approximately 25 minutes.

5. Garnish with chopped parsley and green bell pepper.

Rich in the following Antioxidant Nutrients:

Vitamin A	Beta Carotene
Vitamin C	Alpha Carotene
Vitamin E	Lycopene

Plant Antioxidants:

Olive Oil
Oregano
Garlic
Paprika
Onion
Tabasco
Green Bell Pepper
Tomatoes
Red Bell Pepper

To enhance antioxidant quotient, add the following: After cooking, add sliced fresh tomatoes and fresh chopped basil to the dish as a garnish.

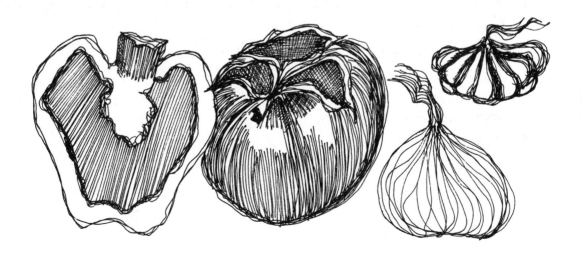

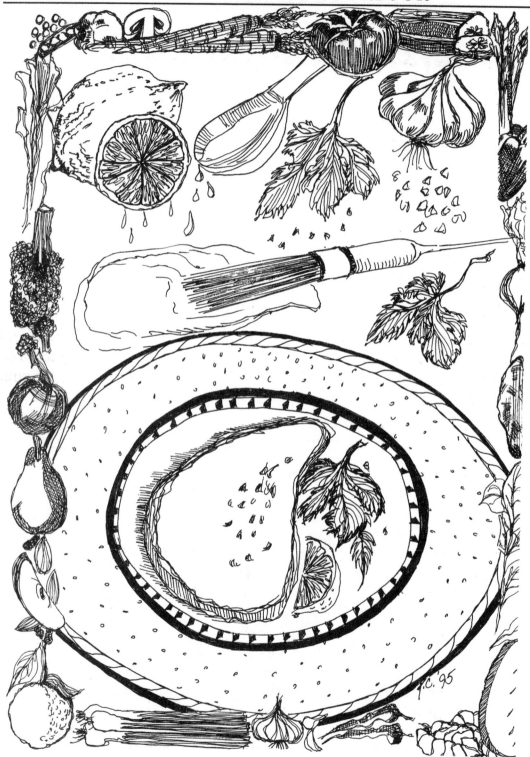

CILANTRO CHICKEN

4   boneless, skinless chicken breast halves, pounded into 3/4″ filets
2   tablespoons lime juice
1   tablespoon honey
1/2   cup (unseasoned) bread crumbs
2   teaspoons fresh minced garlic
3   tablespoons fresh chopped cilantro
1/4   cup safflower oil

1. Combine honey and lime juice

2. Coat chicken breasts with honey/lime mixture. Coat with bread crumbs.

3. Heat safflower oil in 12″ sauté pan over medium heat. Cook chicken and garlic in butter — approximately 3 minutes — on each side (each side having browned). Then cook until done (when meat is no longer pink inside).

4. Garnish with chopped fresh cilantro.

Rich in the following Antioxidant Nutrients:

Vitamin A	Beta Carotene
Vitamin C	Alpha Carotene
Vitamin E	Lycopene

Plant Antioxidants:

Safflower Oil
Garlic
Cilantro
Lime (Citrus Bioflavonoids)

To enhance antioxidant quotient, add the following: After cooking, add fresh papaya, apples, or mango slices to the top of the chicken.

CRAB CAKES

1	pound cooked crab meat
1½	cups bread crumbs
2	medium scallions (green onions), minced
2	tablespoons minced carrot (½ small carrot)
1	egg white
2	teaspoons fresh minced garlic
2	teaspoons fresh lemon juice
1	teaspoon Worcester sauce
½	teaspoon white pepper
½	cup plain low fat yogurt
2	tablespoons water
¼	cup fresh chopped parsley
2	tablespoons peanut oil

1. Whisk together ¼ cup yogurt, garlic, lemon juice, Worcester sauce and pepper. Set aside.

2. Toss the crab meat with ½ cup bread crumbs, carrots, scallions and egg white.

3. Combine the two mixtures. Form into 12 4" round patties (approximately ½" thick). Set aside on a sheet of wax paper.

4. In a shallow bowl stir together remaining yogurt and water, until you have a liquid consistency.

5. Dip patties in yogurt, then into (remaining) bread crumbs.

6. Brush sauté pan with oil. Cook patties, at medium heat, until browned on each side (approximately 2 minutes per side).

Rich in the following Antioxidant Nutrients:

Vitamin A	Beta Carotene
Vitamin C	Alpha Carotene
Vitamin E	Lycopene

Plant Antioxidants:

Scallions
Carrots
Garlic
Lemon (Citrus Bioflavonoids)
Worcester Sauce
Pepper
Parsley
Peanut Oil

To enhance antioxidant quotient, add the following: After cooking ,add fresh lemon juice, fresh grated carrot, and fresh chopped parsley to tops of crab cakes.

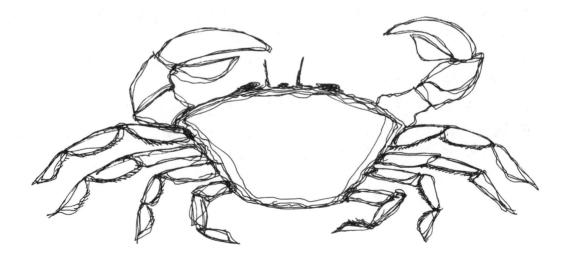

QUICHE, CRUSTLESS VEGETARIAN

1   pound fresh spinach, (or one 10 ounce package frozen
      spinach, defrosted with liquid pressed out) chopped
2   medium white onions, thinly sliced
2   teaspoons olive oil
1/4 teaspoon nutmeg
1/2 pound (fat reduced) swiss cheese, grated
3   eggs
2   tablespoons water

1. Brush large glass pie plate with some of the oil.

2. Brush large sauté pan with oil. Sauté onions until translucent. Add spinach to onions. Heat for 2 additional minutes.

3. Put half of the spinach/onion mixture into the pie plate. Evenly distribute the cheese over spinach. Cover with remaining spinach.

4. Beat eggs, nutmeg and water together in mixing bowl. Pour over spinach. Bake in preheated 400 degree oven for 30 minutes. Let rest 10 minutes before serving.

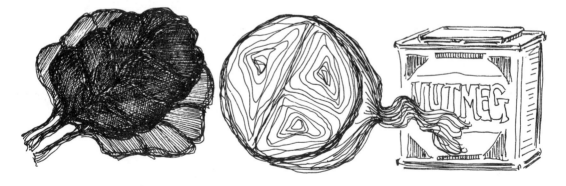

Rich in the following Antioxidant Nutrients:

Vitamin A	Beta Carotene
Vitamin C	Alpha Carotene
Vitamin E	Lycopene

Plant Antioxidants:
Spinach
Onions
Olive Oil
Nutmeg

To enhance antioxidant quotient, add the following: After cooking, garnish with fresh thin red Bermuda onion slices, then top with fresh chopped tomatoes and cilantro.

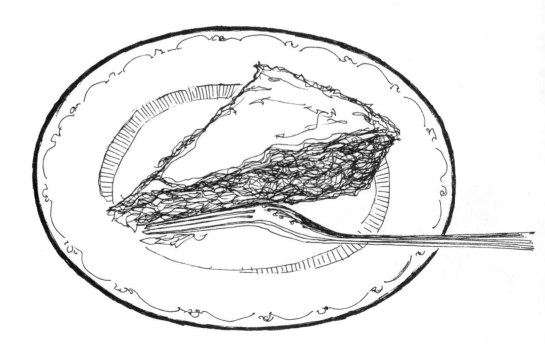

CURRIED CHICKEN

2	pounds boneless, skinless chicken thighs, cut into 2″ strips (approximately 3½ pounds of chicken before boning and skinning.
1	tablespoon safflower oil
2	medium white onions finely chopped
1	tablespoon minced garlic
2	medium tomatoes, chopped
3	tablespoons curry powder
½	cup water
½	cup raisins
2	apples, peeled, cored and sliced
1	tablespoon Italian parsley, chopped for garnish

1. Coat chicken with 1 tablespoon of the curry powder.

2. Brush dutch oven with oil. Heat. Brown chicken on all sides. Remove to a small bowl.

3. Add garlic and onion and apples to the pan. Heat until lightly browned. Stir in curry powder. Cook for an additional minute.

4. Stir in tomato and water cook 1 minute. Add chicken and raisins, and bring to a boil.

5. Lower heat, cover and simmer for 20 minutes. Serve over cous-cous.

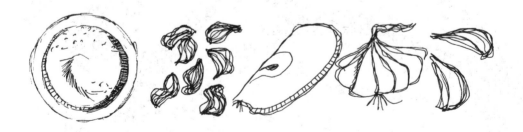

Rich in the following Antioxidant Nutrients:

Vitamin A	Beta Carotene
Vitamin C	Alpha Carotene
Vitamin E	Lycopene

Plant Antioxidants:

Curry Powder
Raisins
Apples
Parsley, Italian
Safflower Oil
Onions
Garlic
Tomatoes

To enhance antioxidant quotient, add the following: After cooking, add fresh apple slices as a garnish.

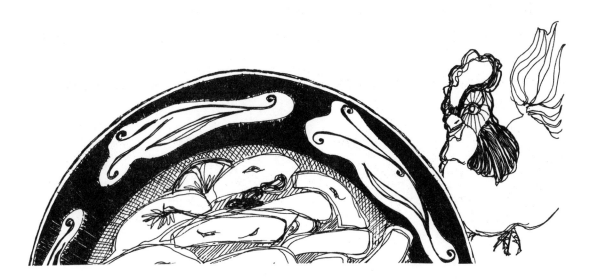

CURRIED SCALLOPS

1/2	medium minced onion
2	teaspoons minced garlic
2	tablespoons chili paste (sauce)
2	tablespoons fresh cilantro
1	tablespoon curry powder
1	teaspoon lemon peel
13	ounces coconut milk
2	teaspoons paprika
1	pound small scallops
3	scallions, cut at a slant
1/2	medium mango, cut into medium dice

1. Combine coconut milk, onion, garlic, chili paste, cilantro, curry powder, lemon peel and paprika in a medium saucepan. Bring to a boil. Lower heat and simmer until slightly thickened.

2. Add scallops. Simmer until scallops are cooked.

3. Stir in mango and scallions. Serve over egg noodles or cellophane noodles.

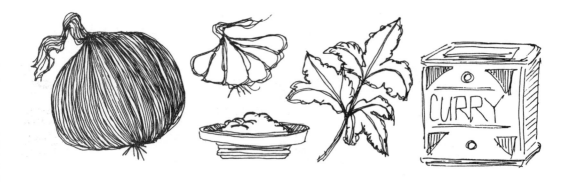

Rich in the following Antioxidant Nutrients:

Vitamin A	Beta Carotene
Vitamin C	Alpha Carotene
Vitamin E	Lycopene

Plant Antioxidants:

Onion
Garlic
Chili Paste
Cilantro
Curry Powder
Lemon Peel
Paprika
Scallions
Mango

To enhance antioxidant quotient, add the following: After cooking, add fresh mango slices and fresh chopped scallions as a garnish.

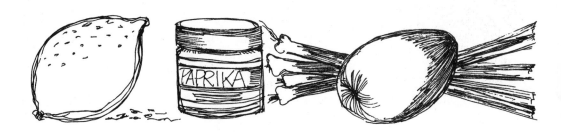

VEGETARIAN DEEP DISH PIZZA
WITH LOW FAT CHEESE

Note for non-vegetarians: Turkey sausage or lemon-pepper sausage may be added.

Crust: See recipe for "No Oil Pie Crust," prepare crust and press into large, shallow glass pie plate.

Filling:

2	teaspoons cornstarch, dissolved in 2 teaspoons water
3	medium tomatoes, peeled seeded and chopped
1	teaspoon olive oil
1/2	medium bermuda onion, finely chopped
2	tablespoons minced garlic
3/4	teaspoon dry basil
3/4	teaspoon oregano
1	teaspoon honey
1/2	teaspoon white pepper
1/2	cup Parmesan cheese, grated
1/2	cup low fat mozzarella cheese, shredded
1/2	red pepper, julienne
2	(turkey) Italian or lemon-pepper sausages, boiled, cut into 1/2" slices (optional)

1. Puree one of the chopped tomatoes together with the basil, oregano, honey and white pepper. Remove to medium size bowl.

2. Sauté onion and garlic in olive oil. Add remaining tomatoes, tomato puree mixture and cornstarch/water mixture. Bring to a boil. Lower heat and allow to simmer for 5 minutes.

3. Spread half of mixture into prepared pie plate. Put in cheeses. Spread remaining filling onto cheese. Bake in preheated 400 degree oven for approximately 15 minutes.

Rich in the following Antioxidant Nutrients:

Vitamin A	Beta Carotene
Vitamin C	Alpha Carotene
Vitamin E	Lycopene

Plant Antioxidants:

Tomatoes
Olive Oil
Bermuda Onion
Garlic
Basil
Oregano
Pepper
Red Bell Pepper

To enhance antioxidant quotient, add the following: After cooking, add fresh chopped basil or oregano or dried chili flakes over pizza.

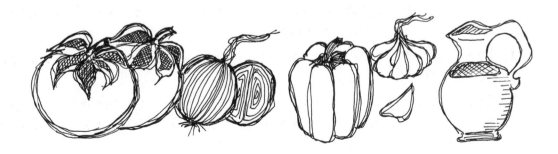

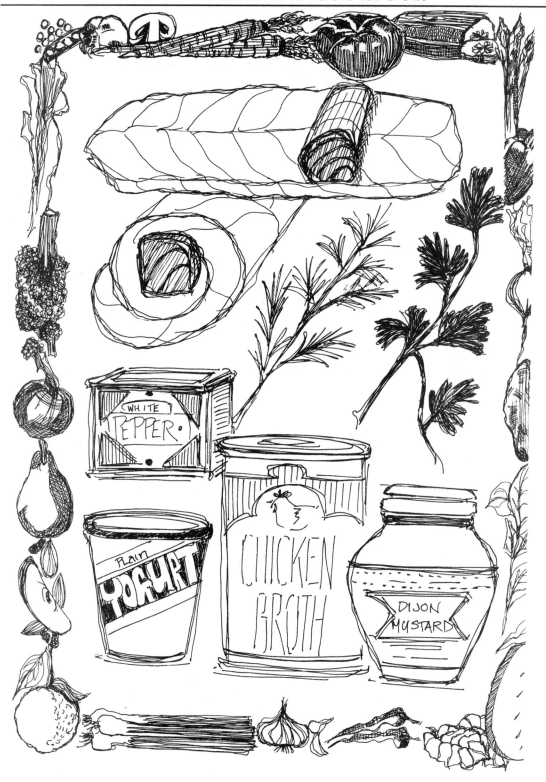

DILL FISH ROLLS

4	flounder filets (4 ounces each)
1	salmon filet (4 to 6 ounces), cut, lengthwise into 4 pieces
1	teaspoon chopped Italian parsley
2	tablespoons chopped fresh dill
1/2	teaspoon white pepper
1/2	cup chicken broth (or 1/2 cup fish stock, page 205)
2	tablespoons plain yogurt
1/2	teaspoon dijon style mustard

1. Spread out flounder filets. Sprinkle with dill and pepper. Place one piece of salmon on the wide end of the flounder filet. roll up, beginning at the wide end and secure roll with a toothpick.

2. Bring broth to a boil in sauté pan. Add fish rolls. Lower heat and simmer, covered, for 8 to 10 minutes. Remove to warm serving plate.

3. To hot broth, remaining in pan, whisk in yogurt and mustard into remaining liquid. Spoon over fish rolls.

Rich in the following Antioxidant Nutrients:

Vitamin A	Beta Carotene
Vitamin C	Alpha Carotene
Vitamin E	Lycopene

Plant Antioxidants:
Parsley, Italian
Dill, Fresh
Pepper
Mustard

To enhance antioxidant quotient, add the following: After cooking, add fresh lemon slices and fresh chopped dill on completed fish rolls.

EGGPLANT LASAGNA

4	large lasagna noodles
1	large eggplant, cut into 2″ cubes
2	medium zucchini sliced to 1/2″ thickness
1	medium white onion, sliced
1	red bell pepper, seeded, cored and sliced
2	cups tomatoes chopped
1/2	cup apple vinegar
2	tablespoons minced garlic
2	teaspoons dried basil
1	teaspoon dried oregano
1/2	teaspoon white pepper
3	cups shredded, low fat mozzarella cheese

1. Cook noodles, al dente. Rinse, set aside

2. Steam eggplant, zucchini, onion and bell pepper for approximately 5 - 7 minutes. Place into a large mixing bowl.

3. Add garlic, basil, tomatoes and oregano to the vegetables.

4. Spread half of this mixture in a 12″ x 7½″ glass baking dish. Top with half of the cheese and the noodles.

5. Add the rest of the vegetables and top with cheese. Bake at 375 degrees for 25 minutes.

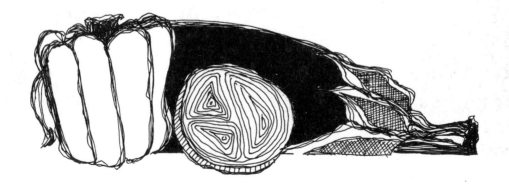

Rich in the following Antioxidant Nutrients:

Vitamin A	Beta Carotene
Vitamin C	Alpha Carotene
Vitamin E	Lycopene

Plant Antioxidants:

Eggplant
Zucchini
Onion
Red Bell Pepper
Tomatoes
Apple Vinegar
Garlic
Basil
Oregano
Pepper

To enhance antioxidant quotient, add the following: After cooking, add slices of fresh red bell pepper as a garnish.

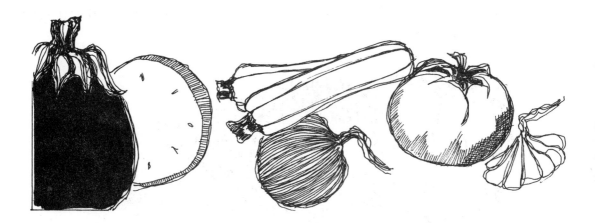

FISH STEW

2	medium white onions, chopped
6	medium tomatoes, peeled, seeded and chopped
1	tablespoon minced garlic
4	cups fish stock*
3/4	teaspoon dried basil
1/2	teaspoon white pepper
3	medium zucchini, cut into 3/4" slices
1	pound red snapper, halibut or shark, cut into 2" pieces
1	red bell pepper, chopped
1	teaspoon olive oil

1. Brush inside of large saucepan with oil. Sauté onions for approximately 3 minutes. Add garlic, sauté an additional minute.

2. Add in tomatoes, fish stock, red bell pepper, zucchini, basil, thyme and pepper. Cover and simmer for 10 minutes.

3. Add fish pieces. Simmer 5 to 7 minutes until fish is done.

* Fish Stock recipe page 205, or buy freeze dried packets that may be reconstituted with water.

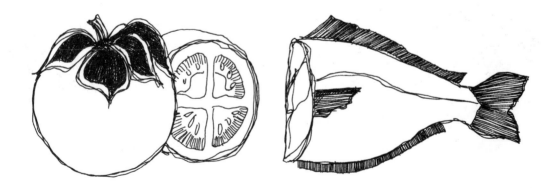

Rich in the following Antioxidant Nutrients:

Vitamin A	Beta Carotene
Vitamin C	Alpha Carotene
Vitamin E	Lycopene

Plant Antioxidants:

Onion
Tomatoes
Garlic
Basil
Oregano
Pepper
Red Bell Pepper
Olive Oil

To enhance antioxidant quotient, add the following: After cooking, add fresh sliced carrots.

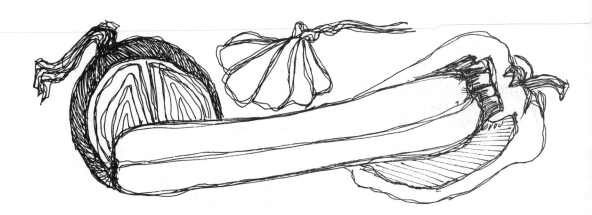

FRITATTA WITH TURKEY OR CHICKEN SAUSAGE

1/2	pound turkey or chicken sausage
1	medium white onion, chopped
1	medium tomato, peeled, seeded and chopped
1	russet potato, peeled and grated
1	tablespoon olive oil
2	teaspoons Italian parsley, chopped
1	teaspoon dry chopped basil
2	teaspoons minced garlic
3	eggs
1	red bell pepper
2	tablespoons water

1. Brown sausage. Drain all fat.

2. Brush sauté pan with olive oil. Add onions and garlic. Cook until translucent.

3. Add potatoes and red bell pepper. Cook for an additional 3 minutes.

4. Remove from heat. Add tomato, parsley and basil.

5. Brush a large, shallow casserole dish with remaining oil. Place mixture into the dish.

5. In a small bowl beat the eggs and water until foamy. Pour over mixture. Bake in preheated 370 degree oven for 30 minutes, in covered casserole dish.

Rich in the following Antioxidant Nutrients:

Vitamin A	Beta Carotene
Vitamin C	Alpha Carotene
Vitamin E	Lycopene

Plant Antioxidants:

Basil
Garlic
Red Bell Pepper
Onion
Olive Oil
Tomato
Parsley, Italian

To enhance antioxidant quotient, add the following: After cooking, add fresh apples slices, fresh chopped basil, and fresh chopped parsley as a garnish.

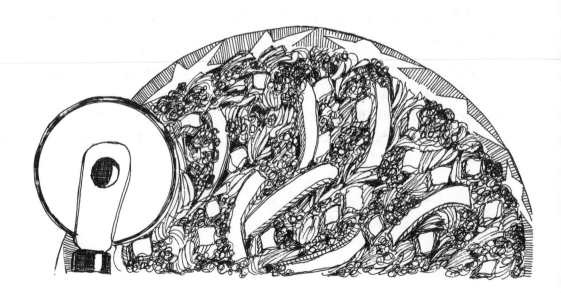

FRITATTA, VEGETARIAN

2   eggplants, Japanese, slice lengthwise
1   medium white onion, chopped
1   medium tomato, peeled, seeded and chopped
1   russet potato, peeled and grated
1   tablespoon olive oil
2   teaspoons Italian parsley, chopped
1   teaspoon dry chopped basil
2   teaspoons minced garlic
3   eggs
1   red bell pepper
2   tablespoons water

1. Brown sliced eggplant in olive oil. Cut into 1" pieces.

2. Brush sauté pan with olive oil. Add onions and garlic. Cook until translucent.

3. Add potatoes and red bell pepper. Cook for an additional 3 minutes.

4. Remove from heat. Add tomato, parsley and basil.

5. Brush a large, shallow casserole dish with remaining oil. Place eggplant, potatoes, and red bell pepper into the dish.

5. In a small bowl beat the eggs and water until mixture is foamy. Pour over casserole contents. Bake in preheated 370 degree oven for 30 minutes, uncovered.

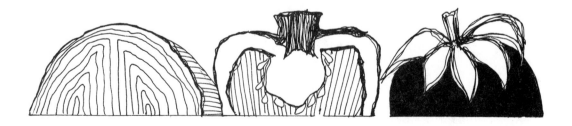

Rich in the following Antioxidant Nutrients:

Vitamin A	Beta Carotene
Vitamin C	Alpha Carotene
Vitamin E	Lycopene

Plant Antioxidants:

Basil
Garlic
Red Bell Pepper
Onion
Olive Oil
Tomato
Parsley, Italian
Eggplant, Japanese

To enhance antioxidant quotient, add the following: After cooking, add sliced fresh tomatoes and ground pepper or cayenne pepper to the top of the fritatta.

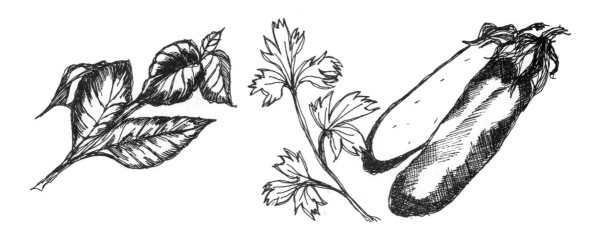

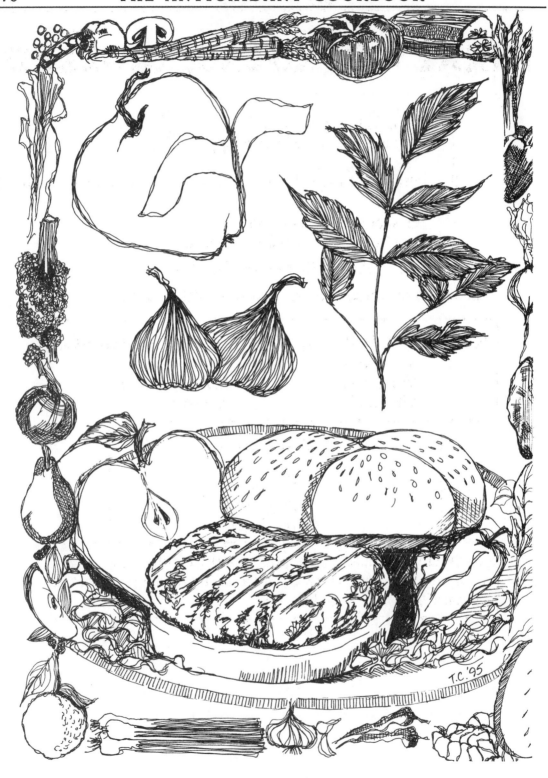

TURKEY BURGERS, GRILLED

1½   pounds lean ground turkey
1   apple peeled, cored and chopped
1   egg
2   shallots, finely chopped (¼ white onion may be substituted
     here)
¼   teaspoon ground oregano
¼   cup fresh Italian parsley, chopped

1. Combine all ingredients. Shape into 3″ sized patties.
2. Grill patties over medium heat. Garnish with parsley.

Rich in the following Antioxidant Nutrients:

Vitamin A	Beta Carotene
Vitamin C	Alpha Carotene
Vitamin E	Lycopene

Plant Antioxidants:
Apple
Shallots
Oregano
Parsley, Italian

To enhance antioxidant quotient, add the following: After cooking, add fresh grated carrot and cabbage and fresh tomato slices to turkey burgers.

GUMBO

4	cups steamed rice
2	tablespoons olive oil
3	medium zucchini, cut into 1" slices
1	tablespoon minced garlic
1	large white onion, chopped
4	cups Fish Stock (Sea Bags are an excellent product to use here or see Fish Stock recipe, page 205)
4	medium tomatoes, peeled, seeded and chopped
1	teaspoon gumbo file (found in specialty stores)
1/8	teaspoon chili flakes
8	ounces medium shrimp, in shells
4	turkey (Italian) sausages, boiled, cut into 1" slices
1	pound chicken, boneless and skinless cut into 1" pieces

1. Heat oil in 5 quart heavy pot. Add in onion and garlic. Sauté until lightly browned.

2. Add fish stock, tomatoes, gumbo file and chili flakes, bring to a boil. Lower heat and simmer for 10 minutes.

3. Add chicken and zucchini. Cover and simmer for 10 additional minutes.

4. Add sausage and shrimp. Cover and simmer for 3 to 4 more minutes. Serve in bowls over scoops of steamed rice.

Rich in the following Antioxidant Nutrients:

Vitamin A   Beta Carotene
Vitamin C   Alpha Carotene
Vitamin E   Lycopene

Plant Antioxidants:

Olive Oil
Zucchini
Garlic
Onion
Tomatoes
Chili Flakes

To enhance antioxidant quotient, add the following: After cooking, add fresh grated ginger and fresh sliced red pepper.

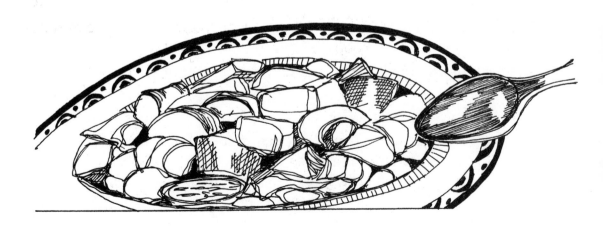

LEMON CHICKEN SAUSAGE WHOLE WHEAT PITA POCKETS

Filling:

1½	pound lemon-chicken sausage — very lean
1	medium white onion, finely chopped
2	teaspoons fresh minced garlic
1	teaspoon parsley, minced
1	teaspoon fresh lemon juice
1	teaspoon white pepper
1	egg white
3	large whole wheat pita pockets, halved
1	tablespoon safflower oil
2	medium tomatoes, sliced
6	large lettuce leaves

1. Combine cooked chopped lemon-chicken sausage, onion, garlic, parsley, lemon juice, pepper and egg white. Roll into 18 meatballs.

2. Brush sauté pan with oil. Cook meatballs until brown. Approximately 10 minutes.

3. Line pita halves with lettuce. add tomatoes and meatballs.

Dressing:

4	ounces plain yogurt
½	medium cucumber, peeled, seeded, finely chopped
1	teaspoon lemon juice
½	teaspoon mint leaves (fresh or dried)

1. Combine all ingredients. Spoon onto filled pockets.

Rich in the following Antioxidant Nutrients:

Vitamin A	Beta Carotene
Vitamin C	Alpha Carotene
Vitamin E	Lycopene

Plant Antioxidants:

Safflower Oil

Tomatoes

Lettuce

Cucumber

Mint

Onion

Garlic or Parsley, Fresh

Lemon (Citrus Bioflavonoid)

Pepper

To enhance antioxidant quotient, add the following: After preparing, garnish with fresh cucumber slices and mint leaves.

LASAGNA ROLL UPS

6   lasagna noodles, cooked al dente, rinsed in cold water
1/2   pound spinach, stemmed, steamed, water pressed out. (If frozen, defrost and press out as much of the liquid as you can.) Chop.
1   cup part-skimmed ricotta cheese
2   tablespoons grated Parmesan cheese
1/2   teaspoon dry fresh basil
8   ounces tomato sauce — see below

1. Combine ingredients.

2. Place on equal amounts on end of noodle and roll up.

3. Place upright in small casserole. Pour sauce around rolls. Bake in preheated oven, at 425 degrees for 20 minutes.

Sauce:

4   medium tomatoes, peeled and diced
4   scallions, minced
1   tablespoon chopped fresh basil
1   tablespoon apple cider vinegar
1   teaspoon minced garlic
1/2   medium white onion, thinly sliced
1   teaspoon olive oil
2   teaspoons chopped cilantro, to garnish

1. Brush sauté pan with oil. Sauté onion and garlic until soft.

2. Add all other ingredients. Bring to a boil, lower heat. Simmer for 10 minutes, or longer, to taste.

Rich in the following Antioxidant Nutrients:

Vitamin A   Beta Carotene
Vitamin C   Alpha Carotene
Vitamin E   Lycopene

Plant Antioxidants:

Tomatoes
Scallions
Basil
Apple Cider Vinegar
Garlic
Onion
Olive Oil
Cilantro, Fresh

To enhance antioxidant quotient, add the following: After cooking ,add fresh grated zucchini and ground black pepper to top of lasagna.

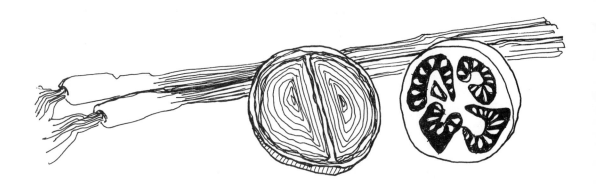

LAVASH I VEGETARIAN
MIDDLE-EASTERN SANDWICH

Once you know how to prepare the bread you will come up with any number of fillings of your own.

1   large round lavash (found in specialty stores and some large supermarkets)
4   ounces low fat cream cheese
1/4 cup fresh basil, minced
1/4 cup toasted pine nuts
2   medium tomatoes, thinly sliced

* You will need two medium cloth kitchen towels, dampened

1. Moisten lavash well on both sides under cold running water. Put lavash between the towels and set aside until pliable, approximately 30 minutes.

2. Combine cream cheese, basil and pine nuts.

3. Take off top towel. Trim the lavash to create a square sheet.

4. Spread the cream cheese mixture onto the lavash, leaving a 2" margin on one side. Top this with a layer of tomatoes.

5. Roll the sheet, beginning with marginate edge, in jelly roll fashion. Cover and chill until ready to serve. I recommend this be made a day ahead. Slice into 1" sections when ready to serve.

Rich in the following Antioxidant Nutrients:

Vitamin A	Beta Carotene
Vitamin C	Alpha Carotene
Vitamin E	Lycopene

Plant Antioxidants:

Basil
Tomatoes
Pine Nuts

To enhance antioxidant quotient, add the following: After preparing, add chopped black olives and chopped pine nuts over lavash.

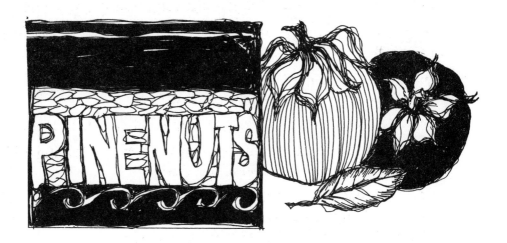

LAVASH II

See directions for bread in Lavash I

Filling:

1	eggplant slice into ½″ thick slices, lengthwise
1	cup roasted red pepper (oil and juice drained)
2	medium tomatoes, thinly sliced
1	teaspoon paprika
1	teaspoon cumin
2	tablespoons lemon juice
1	tablespoon minced garlic
½	cup fresh Italian parsley, chopped
1	ounce olive oil
	salt to taste

1. Brush eggplant, lightly with olive oil on both sides. Place on baking sheet at 450 degrees for 15 minutes. Cool.

2. Combine eggplant, peppers and garlic in food processor. Process briefly. The texture should be coarse.

3. Remove to a bowl. Stir in paprika, cumin, salt and lemon juice to taste.

4. Spread on lavash. Top with layer of tomato and parsley leaves.

5. Roll and slice into 1″ sections, after chilling in refrigerator for one hour.

Dressing:

1	tablespoon sesame oil
½	cup plain yogurt
¼	cup fresh lemon juice
1	teaspoon minced garlic
½	teaspoon ground cumin
1	tablespoon honey
	salt to taste

1. Whisk together all ingredients. Cover and refrigerate for 30 minutes before use.

Rich in the following Antioxidant Nutrients:

Vitamin A   Beta Carotene
Vitamin C   Alpha Carotene
Vitamin E   Lycopene

Plant Antioxidants:

Lemon (Citrus Bioflavonoid
Garlic
Parsley, Italian
Olive Oil
Red Bell Pepper
Tomatoes
Paprika
Cumin

To enhance antioxidant quotient, add the following: After preparing, add fresh chopped Italian parsley, ground paprika, and ground cumin to taste over lavash.

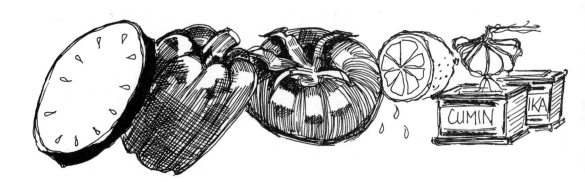

LEMON CHICKEN

4	boneless, skinless chicken breasts
1½	cups long grain rice
3	cups chicken, or vegetable broth, heated
2	teaspoons lemon juice
2	teaspoons lemon peel
½	teaspoon pepper
½	medium white onion, finely chopped
2	teaspoons safflower oil, to coat pan
	chopped parsley to garnish

1. Brush a large dutch oven with oil. Brown chicken on both sides, 3 minutes each side. Remove from pan and set aside.

2. Brush dutch oven with a little more oil. Sauté onion and rice.

3. Add hot broth, rice, lemon juice, and lemon peel. Set chicken breast on top of mixture. Cover.

4. Set into oven, at 325 degrees for 20 minutes. Fluff rice. Garnish with chopped parsley.

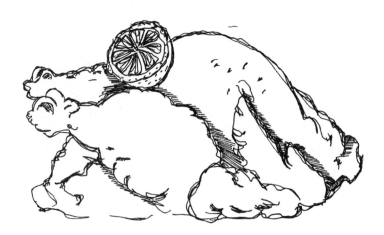

Rich in the following Antioxidant Nutrients:

Vitamin A   Beta Carotene
Vitamin C   Alpha Carotene
Vitamin E   Lycopene

Plant Antioxidants:

Lemon (Citrus Bioflavonoid)
Pepper
Onion
Safflower Oil
Parsley, Fresh

To enhance antioxidant quotient, add the following: After cooking, add fresh lemon and fresh ginger slices over top of chicken.

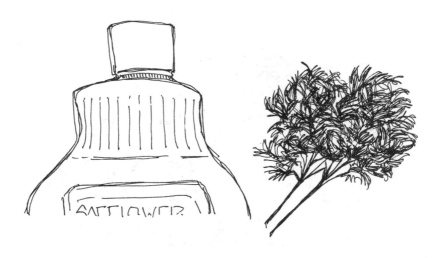

PESTO LINGUINI, VEGETARIAN

12   ounces linguini noodles, cooked al dente, set aside
1/4 cup olive oil
2   cups Italian parsley, chopped
1/4 cup grated Parmesan cheese
1/4 cups toasted walnuts
1/2 dozen fresh basil leaves, chopped
1   clove garlic, minced
1/2 cup chicken broth

1. Cook noodles, al dente.

2. Put all other ingredients in blender. Whirl until smooth. (Scrape the sides down, from time to time while blending. Be certain you turn the blender off before you do this.)

3. Toss the noodles with the pesto.

Rich in the following Antioxidant Nutrients:

Vitamin A	Beta Carotene
Vitamin C	Alpha Carotene
Vitamin E	Lycopene

Plant Antioxidants:

Olive Oil
Parsley, Italian Fresh
Walnuts
Basil, Fresh
Garlic

To enhance antioxidant quotient, add the following: After cooking, add walnut pieces, grated parmesan cheese, and fresh chopped basil to the top of the linguini.

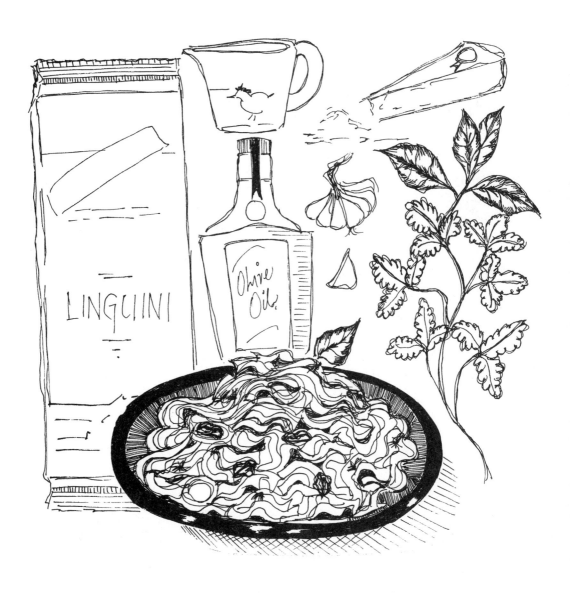

MEATLOAF

(Substitutions: Chicken Loaf, Fish Loaf, Turkey Loaf)

2	pounds extra lean ground beef*
2	eggs
2	teaspoons minced garlic
2	teaspoons chili paste
2/3	cup crushed corn flakes
1/2	teaspoon dried oregano
1	large red or yellow bell pepper, pureed

1. Place all ingredients in a mixing bowl and work, with hands, until all ingredients are well incorporated.

2. Form into a loaf shape. Set onto a rack in a baking dish.

3. Bake in preheated 350 degree oven for approximately 30 to 40 minutes. Let stand 5 minutes before cutting. This can be served hot or cold.

* Substitutions: 2 pounds ground chicken, 2 pounds chopped fish, or 2 pounds ground turkey

Rich in the following Antioxidant Nutrients:

Vitamin A   Beta Carotene

Vitamin C   Alpha Carotene

Vitamin E   Lycopene

Plant Antioxidants:

Garlic

Chili

Oregano

Red or Yellow Bell Pepper

To enhance antioxidant quotient, add the following: After cooking, add fresh chopped basil, fresh chopped tomato, and fresh chopped onion to the top of the meatloaf.

PASTA
WITH
PARMESAN CHEESE
& SPICES

½   pound pasta of choice, cooked al dente
½   cup fresh bread crumbs
½   cup Parmesan cheese, grated
2   tablespoons olive oil
½   cup basil, finely chopped
½   cup Italian parsley, finely chopped
4   scallions, white parts only, sliced
6   cloves garlic, minced
    black fresh ground pepper, to taste

1. Brush pan with oil and sauté and brown bread crumbs over medium heat.
2. Transfer crumbs to bowl. Cool and add Parmesan cheese.
3. Combine the basil, parsley and onions. Toss with remaining oil.
4. Add mixture to noodles. Toss and coat well.
5. Sprinkle with crumb and cheese mixture.
6. Add black fresh ground pepper to taste.

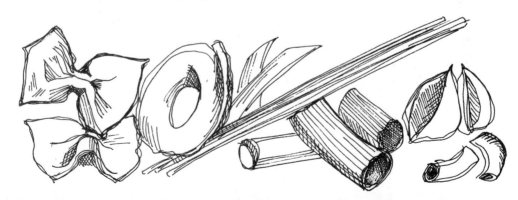

Rich in the following Antioxidant Nutrients:

Vitamin A	Beta Carotene
Vitamin C	Alpha Carotene
Vitamin E	Lycopene

Plant Antioxidants:
Olive Oil
Parsley, Italian Fresh
Scallions
Basil, Fresh
Garlic
Pepper, Black

To enhance antioxidant quotient, add the following: After cooking, add sun-dried tomatoes and fresh minced garlic over the top of the pasta.

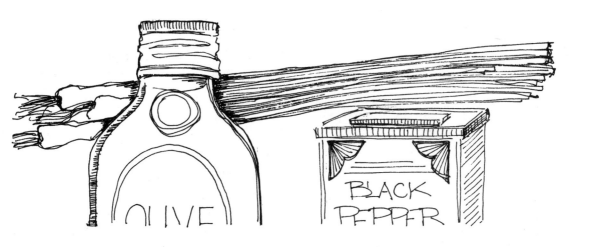

POACHED RED SNAPPER

2	cups steamed white rice
1/2	bermuda onion, chopped
2/3	cup chicken or fish broth (see pages 203 and 205)
1	teaspoon lemon juice
1	teaspoon lemon peel
4	6 ounces red snapper filets
1	tablespoon olive oil
1	medium red bell pepper, chopped
1/4	teaspoon dry tarragon
1	medium zucchini, diced
1	teaspoon minced garlic
1/2	teaspoon minced ginger

1. Combine onion, red pepper, zucchini, chicken broth and lemon juice in large sauté pan. Bring mixture to a boil. Carefully add in snapper filets. Cover and simmer for 6 to 8 minutes until fish flakes.

2. Place bed of hot rice on heated serving plate. With a slotted spoon, spoon vegetables and then fish onto rice. Keep warm.

3. To poaching liquid add oil. Over high heat reduce liquid to approximately 1/4 cup. Remove from heat. Stir in tarragon. Pour over fish.

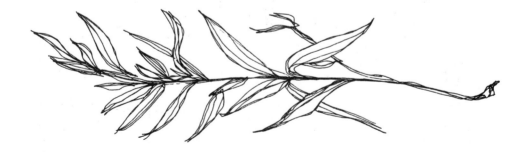

Rich in the following Antioxidant Nutrients:

Vitamin A   Beta Carotene
Vitamin C   Alpha Carotene
Vitamin E   Lycopene

Plant Antioxidants:

Onion, Bermuda
Lemon (Citrus Bioflavonoid)
Olive Oil
Red Bell Pepper
Tarragon
Zucchini
Garlic
Ginger

To enhance antioxidant quotient, add the following: After cooking, add fresh lemon or lime slices, dried tarragon, and fresh ground black pepper over snapper.

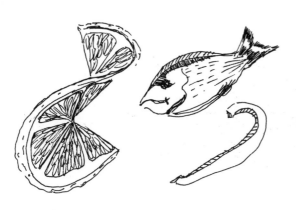

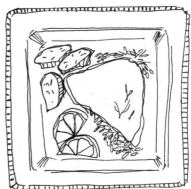

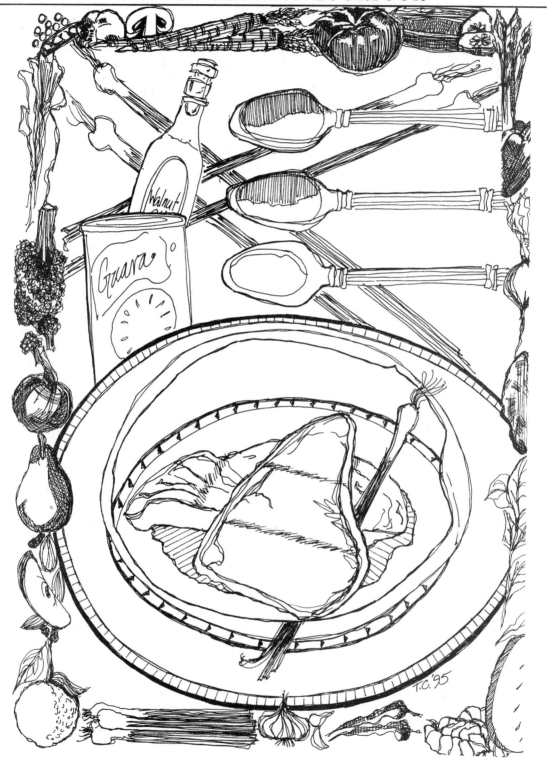

TURKEY BREAST FILETS
WITH GUAVA SAUCE

4   turkey breast filets (2 pounds total)
4   scallions, sliced
1   teaspoon walnut oil
2   teaspoons cornstarch
3/4   cup guava nectar

1. Broil chops, turning once, until done (approximately 20 minutes).

2. In a small saucepan cook green onion in walnut oil, until soft.

3. Combine cornstarch and guava nectar. Add to onions. Bring to a boil, lower heat and simmer for 2 minutes.

4. Pour over broiled filets.

Rich in the following Antioxidant Nutrients:

Vitamin A	Beta Carotene
Vitamin C	Alpha Carotene
Vitamin E	Lycopene

Plant Antioxidants:
Scallions
Walnut Oil
Guava Nectar

To enhance antioxidant quotient, add the following: After cooking, add fresh papaya slices and sun-dried cherries to turkey filets.

CHICKEN & CABBAGE STEW

1   pound lean ground chicken, skinless and boneless
2   medium white onions, chopped
1   tablespoon minced garlic
2   medium tomatoes, peeled and chopped
1   medium apple, cored and chopped
1   teaspoon fresh ginger, grated
½   cup apple cider or juice
2   tablespoons cold water
1   tablespoon cornstarch
½   cup golden raisins
½   head of cabbage, cored and cut into sections

1. In large sauté pan cook chicken, onion and garlic, over medium heat until meat is brown. Drain off any fat.

2. Stir in tomato, apple, apple cider (juice), and ginger. Bring to a boil. Reduce heat, simmer covered for 10 minutes.

3. Combine water and cornstarch. Add to meat mixture. Stir in raisins. Stir constantly until mixture thickens. Let simmer for 2 minutes.

4. At the same time cook cabbage in small amount of boiling water for 10 minutes, or until tender. Drain cabbage sections.

5. Spoon meat mixture over cabbage.

Rich in the following Antioxidant Nutrients:

Vitamin A	Beta Carotene
Vitamin C	Alpha Carotene
Vitamin E	Lycopene

Plant Antioxidants:

Onions
Garlic
Tomatoes
Apple
Ginger
Apple Cider
Raisins
Cabbage

To enhance antioxidant quotient, add the following: After cooking, add fresh apple slices, powdered cinnamon, and powdered nutmeg to taste.

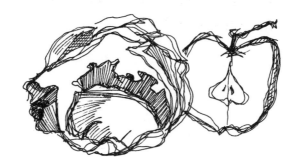

TURKEY STIR SAUTÉ

1	pound lean turkey breast filets, almost frozen, cut into thin slices
3/4	cup orange juice
3	tablespoons (brewed) soy sauce
1/3	cup honey
1	tablespoon corn starch
1	teaspoon fresh ginger, grated
2	teaspoons peanut oil, 1 teaspoon sesame oil, combined
3	scallions, sliced at a slant
2	carrots, sliced diagonally
1	red bell pepper, julienne
1/2	cup unsalted peanuts
1/2	teaspoon chili flakes
1	teaspoon minced garlic

1. Combine orange juice, soy sauce, honey, cornstarch and ginger in a small bowl, mix well.

2. Heat one-half of the oil in large sauté pan, or wok, add carrots and bell pepper. Cook at high heat, approximately 2 minutes. Remove vegetables and set aside.

3. Heat remaining oil in pan. Add garlic and turkey breast filet slices. Stir sauté until done, approximately 3 minutes.

4. Return vegetables to sauté, add sauce mixture and peanuts. Bring mixture to a boil. Lower heat, simmer until sauce thickens. Add scallions before serving. Serve over hot steamed rice.

Rich in the following Antioxidant Nutrients:

Vitamin A	Beta Carotene
Vitamin C	Alpha Carotene
Vitamin E	Lycopene

Plant Antioxidants:

Orange Juice (Citrus Bioflavonoids)
Soy Sauce
Ginger
Peanut Oil
Scallions
Carrots
Red Bell Pepper
Chili Flakes
Garlic

To enhance antioxidant quotient, add the following: After cooking, add fresh sliced ginger, fresh sliced orange, and unsalted ground peanuts to taste.

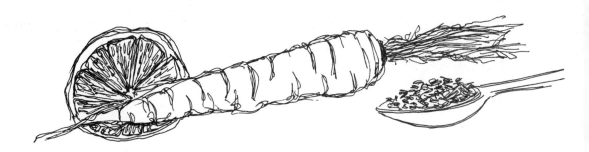

TURGANOFF OR CHICKANOFF
(TURKEY OR CHICKEN STROGANOFF)

8	ounces egg noodles, cooked al dente
1	pound lean turkey breast or chicken breast, cut into strips
3	medium white onions, chopped
2	teaspoons minced garlic
1/2	pound mushrooms, sliced
1/2	cup chicken broth (see page 203)
1	medium tomato, peeled, seeded, chopped
1	teaspoon dry tarragon
1	teaspoon lemon juice
1	teaspoon lemon peel
1/2	cup low fat yogurt
1/4	cup chopped Italian parsley
2	medium carrots, scraped, julienne
1/2	teaspoon white pepper
1	tablespoon olive oil

1. Brush inside of large sauté pan with oil. Heat pan and add turkey or chicken. Stir-fry until done, 3 to 5 minutes. Set aside.

2. Brush inside of sauté pan with additional oil. Add garlic and onion. Sauté for 3 minutes. Add mushrooms, carrots and sauté for an additional 4 minutes.

3. Add chicken broth, tomato, tarragon, lemon juice, lemon peel and pepper, simmer for 5 minutes. Add cooked turkey or chicken to pan, simmering for 2 minutes. Remove from heat.

4. In a small bowl combine yogurt and parsley, combine with chicken or turkey mixture. Serve immediately over small bed of egg noodles.

Rich in the following Antioxidant Nutrients:

Vitamin A	Beta Carotene
Vitamin C	Alpha Carotene
Vitamin E	Lycopene

Plant Antioxidants:

Lemon (Citrus Bioflavonoids)
Parsley, Italian Fresh
Carrots
Pepper
Olive Oil
Onions
Garlic
Mushrooms
Tomato
Tarragon

To enhance antioxidant quotient, add the following: After cooking, add fresh chopped garlic and Italian parsley.

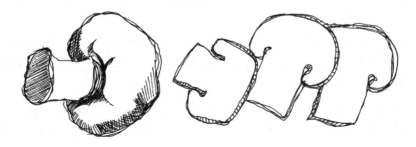

RED SNAPPER FILETS

4	red snapper filets
2	beaten egg whites
1	tablespoon water
1/2	cup bread crumbs
2	tablespoons parsley finely chopped
1	teaspoon white pepper
2	teaspoons minced garlic
1	teaspoon safflower oil

1. Pat fish filets dry.

2. Combine egg whites and water.

3. Combine bread crumbs, garlic, pepper and parsley.

4. Dip filets into egg mixture, then coat with crumbs. Shake off excess crumbs.

5. Brush sauté pan with oil. Heat.

6. Place fish in hot pan. Cook each side approximately 4 minutes, until browned, and fish flakes easily.

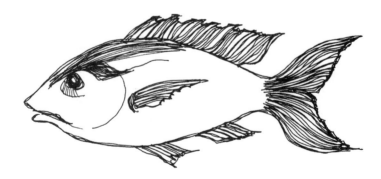

Rich in the following Antioxidant Nutrients:

Vitamin A	Beta Carotene
Vitamin C	Alpha Carotene
Vitamin E	Lycopene

Plant Antioxidants:

Parsley
Pepper
Garlic
Safflower Oil

To enhance antioxidant quotient, add the following: After cooking, add fresh slices of lemon or orange to the top of the fish.

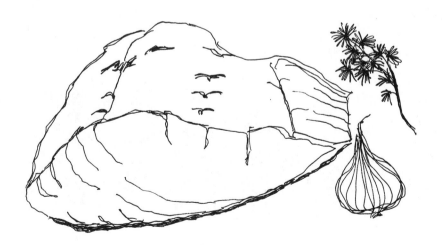

SEAFOOD STIR SAUTÉ

1	pound fresh spinach, (frozen whole leaf spinach may be substituted here, defrosted. All the excess liquid must be pressed out.)
1	each yellow and red bell pepper, cored , seeded and chopped
2	teaspoons minced garlic
1	tablespoon safflower oil
3/4	pound scallops
1/4	pound fresh, cooked crab meat
1	tablespoon lemon juice
1	teaspoon lemon peel
1/4	teaspoon chili flakes

1. Rinse spinach leaves, cut off stems. Hold the leaves in a bunch and cut in half. Set aside.

2. Brush sauté pan with oil. Add peppers and cook for 2 to 3 minutes.

3. Add garlic, scallops, chili flakes, lemon peel and lemon juice. Simmer for 4 to 5 minutes, until centers of scallops are translucent.

4. Stir in spinach. Simmer until spinach is cooked, approximately 4 – 6 minutes. Add in crab. Stir, remove from heat. Serve over cellophane noodles or steamed white rice.

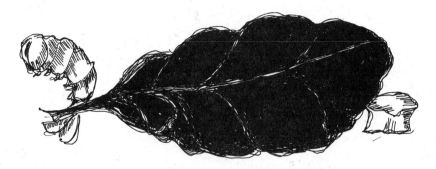

Rich in the following Antioxidant Nutrients:

Vitamin A	Beta Carotene
Vitamin C	Alpha Carotene
Vitamin E	Lycopene

Plant Antioxidants:

Spinach
Yellow Bell Pepper
Red Bell Pepper
Garlic
Safflower Oil
Lemon (Citrus Bioflavonoids)
Chili Flakes

To enhance antioxidant quotient, add the following: After cooking, add sesame seeds, chili flakes, and fresh sliced red pepper as a garnish.

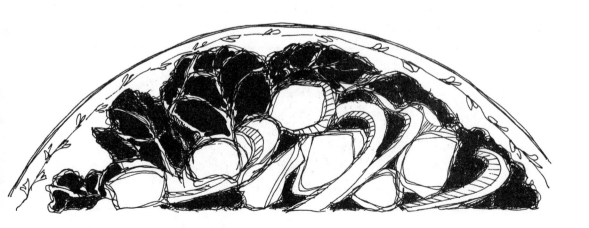

SESAME BROILED SALMON

4	salmon steaks, approximately 6 - 8 ounces each
1/4	cup brewed soy sauce
1/4	cup rice vinegar
1	teaspoon grated fresh ginger
1/4	teaspoon chili paste
1	teaspoon peanut oil
1/2	teaspoon sesame oil
2	teaspoons toasted sesame seeds.

1. Combine all ingredients in large size plastic storage bag.

2. Place salmon steaks in bag. Steaks should be in a single layer, and should marinate for 30 minutes. (Turn the bag periodically to insure both sides of salmon steaks are marinated.)

3. Place salmon steaks under broiler, turn once. (Approximately 4 minutes on each side.)

Rich in the following Antioxidant Nutrients:

Vitamin A	Beta Carotene
Vitamin C	Alpha Carotene
Vitamin E	Lycopene

Plant Antioxidants:

Rice Vinegar
Ginger
Chili Paste
Peanut Oil
Sesame Oil
Sesame Seeds

To enhance antioxidant quotient, add the following: After cooking, add fresh grated ginger, fresh chopped scallions, and toasted sesame seeds as a garnish.

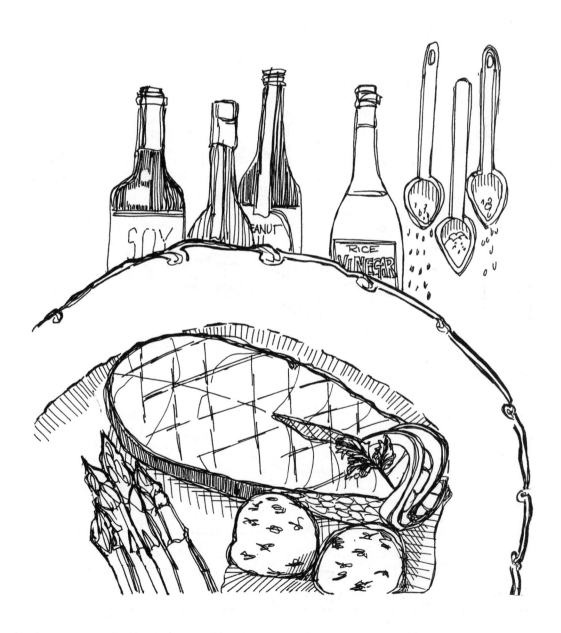

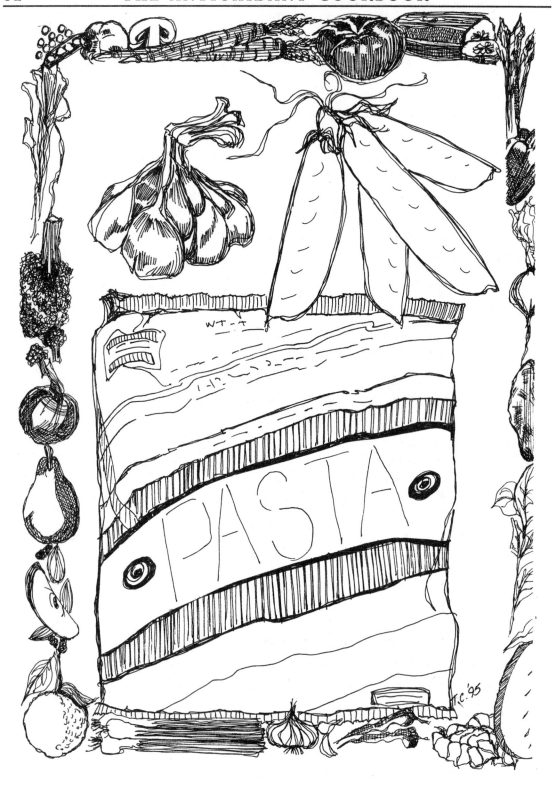

PASTA & SNOW PEAS

2	cups snow peas
4	ounces fettuccine noodles
1	teaspoon safflower oil
1	teaspoon sesame oil
1	teaspoon sesame seeds
½	teaspoon chili paste
½	teaspoon fresh minced garlic

1. Cook noodles in salted boiling water for approximately 6 minutes.

2. Add snow peas to boiling water, with the noodles for one minute. Drain peas and noodles. Rinse with cold water.

3. Combine oils, chili paste and garlic. Add to noodle and pea mixture blend. Sprinkle with sesame seeds.

Rich in the following Antioxidant Nutrients:

Vitamin A	Beta Carotene
Vitamin C	Alpha Carotene
Vitamin E	Lycopene

Plant Antioxidants:

Snow Peas
Safflower Oil
Sesame Seeds
Sesame Oil
Chili Paste
Garlic

To enhance antioxidant quotient, add the following: After cooking, add fresh grated carrot and sliced mango or papaya to pasta.

TACOS, SOFT WITH CHOPPED STEAK*

*(Substitutions: Tofu, Chicken, Fish, or Turkey)

1	pound flank steak*
1	large red onion, thinly sliced
1	red bell pepper, cored, seeded, sliced
1	teaspoon garlic minced
1/4	cup lime juice
1/2	teaspoon lime peel
1	tablespoon olive oil
2	tablespoons cilantro, chopped
1/4	teaspoon ground cumin
2	cups cooked, or 1 14 ounce can cooked pinto beans
1	teaspoon chili paste
1	dozen whole wheat flour tortillas

1. Mix garlic, lime juice, lime peel, oil, cilantro and cumin in a small bowl. Pour over steak, onions and bell pepper. Let stand for 15 minutes.

2. Heat beans in small sauce pan. Drain. Toss with chili paste.

3. Broil steak 2 minutes, on each side. Add onions and bell pepper to the broiling pan. Spoon remaining marinade over the steak and onions and peppers. Broil. Turn several times until steak has reached desired doneness.

4. Allow meat to stand 5 minutes before slicing. Slice, diagonally, into thin strips.

5. Spoon steak, onions, peppers and beans onto warmed tortillas. Fold over.

Rich in the following Antioxidant Nutrients:

Vitamin A	Beta Carotene
Vitamin C	Alpha Carotene
Vitamin E	Lycopene

Plant Antioxidants:

Onion
Red Bell Pepper
Garlic
Lime (Citrus Bioflavonoid)
Olive Oil
Cilantro, Fresh
Cumin
Chili Paste

To enhance antioxidant quotient, add the following: After preparing, add fresh diced papaya or mango slices and tabasco to tacos.

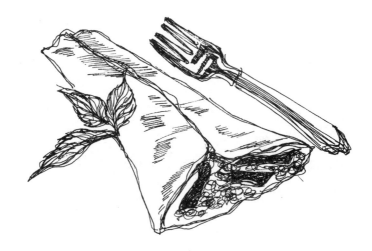

SOUTHWEST CHICKEN

4	boneless, skinless chicken breasts
1	tablespoon chili powder
1	teaspoon pepper
1	teaspoon cumin
1	teaspoon minced garlic
1	medium white onion, chopped
3	medium tomatoes, peeled, quartered
1	red bell pepper, julienne
3	tablespoons walnut oil
	salt to taste

1. Heat walnut oil in 12″ sauté pan — over medium heat, cook chicken until browned, approximately 3 minutes on each side.

2. Remove chicken temporarily.

3. In walnut oil remaining in pan, sauté garlic, onion and red bell pepper. Sauté until tender.

4. Add tomatoes, chili powder, pepper, cumin and salt.

5. Return chicken to pan. Cover, simmer under very low heat until chicken is cooked, 10 - 15 minutes.

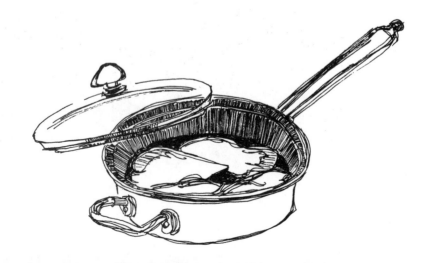

Rich in the following Antioxidant Nutrients:

Vitamin A	Beta Carotene
Vitamin C	Alpha Carotene
Vitamin E	Lycopene

Plant Antioxidants:

Chili Powder
Pepper
Cumin
Garlic
Onion
Tomatoes
Red Bell Pepper
Walnut Oil

To enhance antioxidant quotient, add the following: After cooking, add slices of fresh tomato and ground walnuts to top of dish.

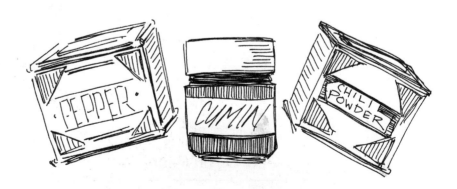

SPINACH CASSEROLE

4	cups cooked spinach (or two 10 ounce packages frozen spinach, cooked and liquid pressed out)
1	medium white onion, minced
1/4	teaspoon white pepper
1/4	teaspoon nutmeg
2	eggs, slightly beaten
1	cup low fat milk
1/2	cup dry bread crumbs, 1/4 parmesan cheese grated — combined
1	teaspoon olive oil or walnut oil

1. Combine spinach, onion pepper and nutmeg.

2. Combine eggs and milk* and add to spinach mixture.

3. Brush oil in baking dish. Pour spinach mixture into dish. Sprinkle with bread crumb and parmesan mixture (bread crumbs, parmesan cheese).

4. Bake in preheated 450 degree oven for approximately 15 minutes or until topping is browned.

Rich in the following Antioxidant Nutrients:

Vitamin A	Beta Carotene
Vitamin C	Alpha Carotene
Vitamin E	Lycopene

Plant Antioxidants:

Spinach
Onion
Pepper
Nutmeg
Olive Oil or Walnut Oil

To enhance antioxidant quotient, add the following: After cooking, add fresh sliced lemons and fresh chopped Italian parsley to casserole.

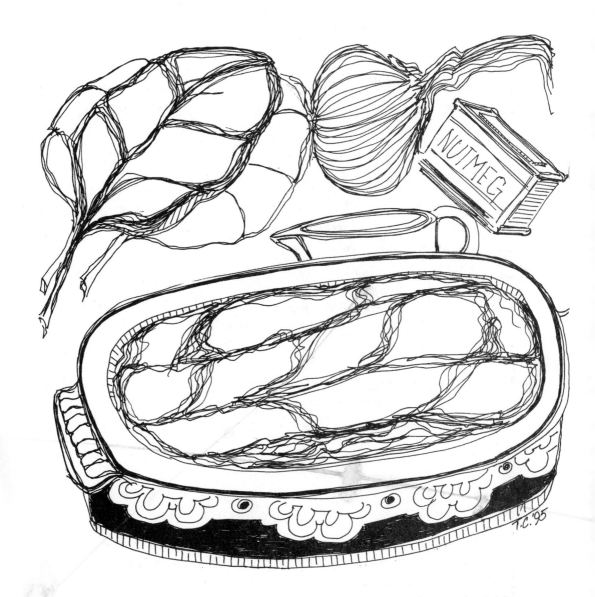

STEAMED (POACHED) FISH
(WITH CITRUS DRESSING)

4	6 ounces red snapper, or halibut filets
1/2	bottle dry white wine
1	medium white onion, thinly sliced
1/2	teaspoon dry dill

1. Preheat oven to 450 degrees

2. Line lasagna sized glass baking dish with onion and dill. Arrange fish filets on top.

3. Pour wine along the side of fish until the fish is 1" deep in the wine. Water may be added if you do not have enough wine.

4. Cover and cook for 10 minutes.

Citrus Dressing:

2/3	cup orange juice
1/4	cup lime juice
1/4	cup lemon juice
1	teaspoon each lime and lemon peel
1	clove garlic, minced
1	teaspoon honey

Combine all ingredients in a small saucepan. Reduce heat; simmer slowly until 1/4 of the liquid has cooked away.

Rich in the following Antioxidant Nutrients:

Vitamin A	Beta Carotene
Vitamin C	Alpha Carotene
Vitamin E	Lycopene

Plant Antioxidants:

White Wine
Onion
Dill, Fresh
Orange Juice (Citrus Limonene)
Lime Juice (Citrus Bioflavonoids)
Garlic

To enhance antioxidant quotient, add the following: After cooking, add fresh grape halves and fresh dill sprigs to the fish.

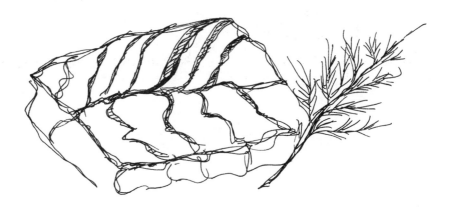

STUFFED CHICKEN LEGS

6	large chicken legs (thigh and drumstick portion) skinned and boned. Set aside.
1	cup unseasoned bread crumbs
1/2	medium white onion, minced
1/2	cup blanched almonds, finely chopped
1/3	cup milk
1	egg, beaten
2	tablespoons walnut oil
1/4	teaspoon ground ginger
1/2	teaspoon cinnamon
1/2	teaspoon nutmeg
1/8	teaspoon dry thyme
1	teaspoon safflower oil, to brush coat the bottom of the baking dish

1. Combine milk and egg in a small bowl

2. Soak crumbs in milk and egg mixture.

3. Add remaining ingredients, except the chicken, and blend thoroughly.

4. Fill the deboned portion of the chicken leg with stuffing. Close openings with toothpicks. Place in oil brushed baking dish.

5. Pour in 3 cups boiling water, enough to fill the pan about 1/2"

6. Cook at 350 degrees approximately 40 minutes or until chicken is tender.

Rich in the following Antioxidant Nutrients:

Vitamin A	Beta Carotene
Vitamin C	Alpha Carotene
Vitamin E	Lycopene

Plant Antioxidants:

Almonds
Onion
Walnut Oil
Ginger
Cinnamon
Nutmeg
Thyme
Safflower Oil

To enhance antioxidant quotient, add the following: After cooking, add fresh grated lemon peel and fresh cherries.

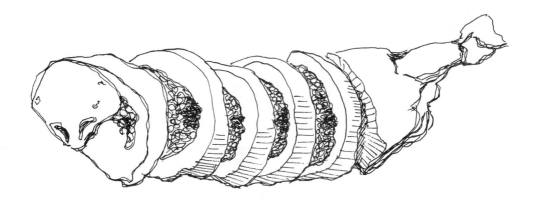

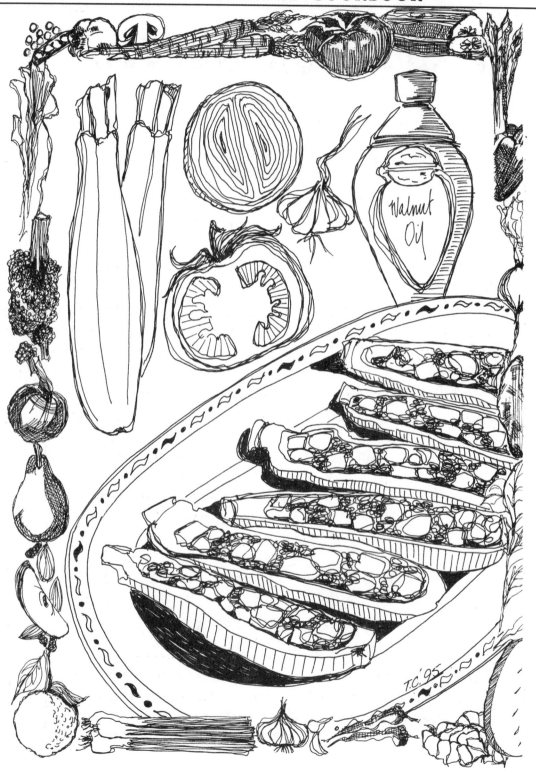

ZUCCHINI, STUFFED

1	tablespoon Italian parsley chopped
2	medium zucchini
2	tablespoons minced onion
1	tablespoon minced garlic
1	cup seasoned bread crumbs
1	tablespoon walnut oil (or peanut oil)
1	medium tomato, peeled and diced

1. Cook whole zucchini in boiling water for 10 minutes. Remove from water.

2. Cut zucchini in halves, lengthwise and scoop out centers. Combine innards with onions, bread crumbs, garlic, tomato and parsley. Spoon mixture into zucchini shells. Bake in preheated 350 degree oven for 15 minutes.

Rich in the following Antioxidant Nutrients:

Vitamin A	Beta Carotene
Vitamin C	Alpha Carotene
Vitamin E	Lycopene

Plant Antioxidants:

Parsley, Italian
Zucchini
Onion
Garlic
Walnut Oil or Peanut Oil
Tomato

To enhance antioxidant quotient, add the following: After cooking, add fresh garlic, oregano, and thyme, and grated parmesan cheese over zucchini.

TAMALE PIE

1	pound lean ground beef
1	teaspoon chili paste
2	cups cooked kidney beans, or pinto beans (1 16 ounce can may be substituted here), drain
2	teaspoons minced garlic
1	teaspoon cumin
1	tablespoon chili flakes
5	corn tortillas
2	cups (reduced fat) cheddar cheese, shredded
6	medium tomatoes, peeled and chopped (1 16 ounce can of Italian tomatoes may be substituted here)
1	4 ounce can chopped green chilies
1	medium white onion, finely chopped
2	teaspoons olive oil

1. Sauté ground beef until browned. Drain fat. Set meat aside.

2. Combine tomatoes, chilies and onions. Combine with ground beef.

3. Combine beans, chili flakes, chili paste and cumin. Coarsely mash with potato masher. Set aside.

4. Brush 8½" round casserole dish with oil.

5. Heat tortillas over open flame very briefly on both sides. Place 3 tortillas along the side and bottom of the dish.

6. Spoon one-third of the bean mixture, one-third of the meat and tomato mixture and one-third of the shredded cheese in layers. Place a single tortilla over these layers and repeat. The last thing on the top layer will be cheese. Bake in preheated 350 degree oven for 30 minutes.

Rich in the following Antioxidant Nutrients:

Vitamin A	Beta Carotene
Vitamin C	Alpha Carotene
Vitamin E	Lycopene

Plant Antioxidants:

Chili Paste & Flakes
Garlic
Cumin
Tomato
Chilies, Green
Onion
Olive Oil

To enhance antioxidant quotient, add the following: After cooking, add fresh chopped onion and cilantro, fresh chopped tomatoes, and minced garlic over tamales.

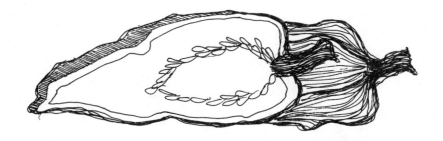

THAI FETTUCINE

8	ounces fettucine noodles, cooked al dente
1	teaspoon minced ginger
1	teaspoon safflower oil, 1 teaspoon sesame oil, combined
2	tablespoons peanut butter
1/2	teaspoon chili paste
1	tablespoon cornstarch
1/2	cup chicken broth (see page 203)
1	tablespoon brewed soy sauce
1	tablespoon rice vinegar
1/2	pound snow peas
1/2	bermuda (red) onion, thinly sliced
3	cloves garlic, finely chopped

1. Cook pasta al dente, set aside

2. Brush sauté pan with oil, sauté garlic, until translucent.

3. Dissolve starch in chicken broth. Combine with peanut butter, chili paste, ginger, soy sauce and vinegar. Pour into sauté pan with garlic. Bring to a boil, Stirring constantly. Lower heat. Simmer until mixture is thickened. Remove from heat.

4. Immediately add snow peas and onions. Toss with noodles.

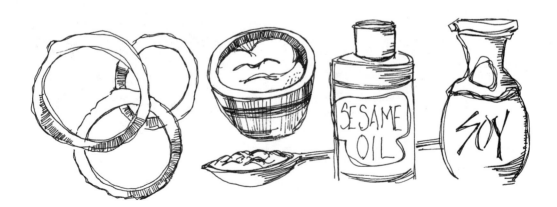

Rich in the following Antioxidant Nutrients:

Vitamin A   Beta Carotene
Vitamin C   Alpha Carotene
Vitamin E   Lycopene

Plant Antioxidants:

Soy Sauce
Ginger
Safflower Oil
Peanut
Chili Paste
Rice Vinegar
Snow Peas
Onion, Bermuda

To enhance antioxidant quotient, add the following: After cooking, add chopped unsalted peanuts and toasted sesame seeds over noodles.

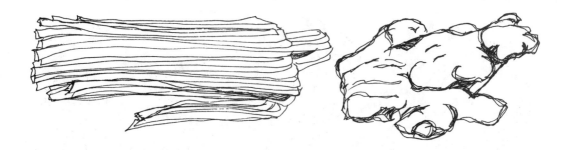

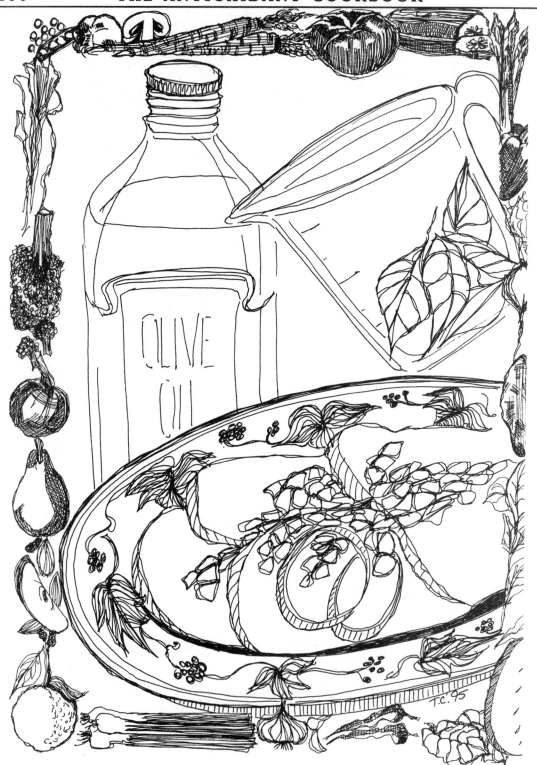

TOMATO BASIL CHICKEN OR TURKEY BREAST

1	teaspoon olive oil
4	lean, skinned, boneless, chicken or turkey breast cutlets pounded to 1/4" thickness
1	medium white onion, minced
3	medium tomatoes, peeled, seeded, chopped
1/4	cup chopped fresh basil
	cayenne pepper to taste

1. Brush sauté pan with oil. Brown poultry cutlets on both sides. Set aside.

2. Sauté onion and garlic until soft. Add in tomatoes. Cook, covered for 10 minutes.

3. Return cutlets to pan, stir in basil. Cover and cook for an additional 5 minutes.

Rich in the following Antioxidant Nutrients:

Vitamin A	Beta Carotene
Vitamin C	Alpha Carotene
Vitamin E	Lycopene

Plant Antioxidants:
Olive Oil
Onion
Tomato
Basil
Pepper, Cayenne

To enhance antioxidant quotient, add the following: Add fresh sliced onions and fresh sliced tomatoes as a garnish.

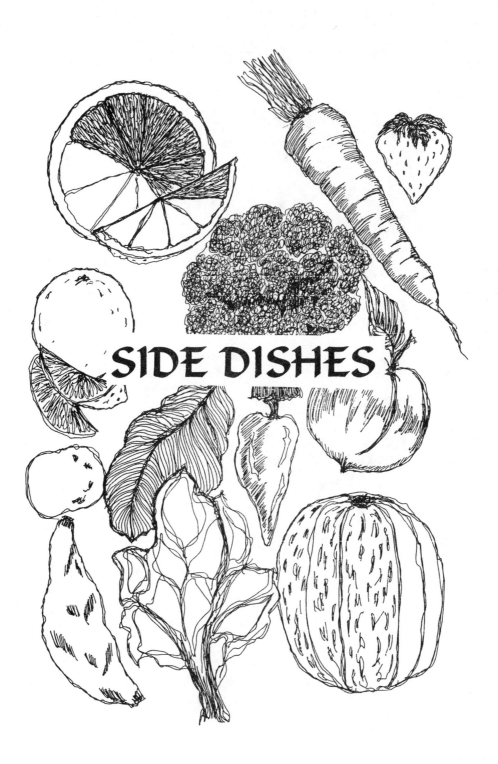

SIDE DISHES

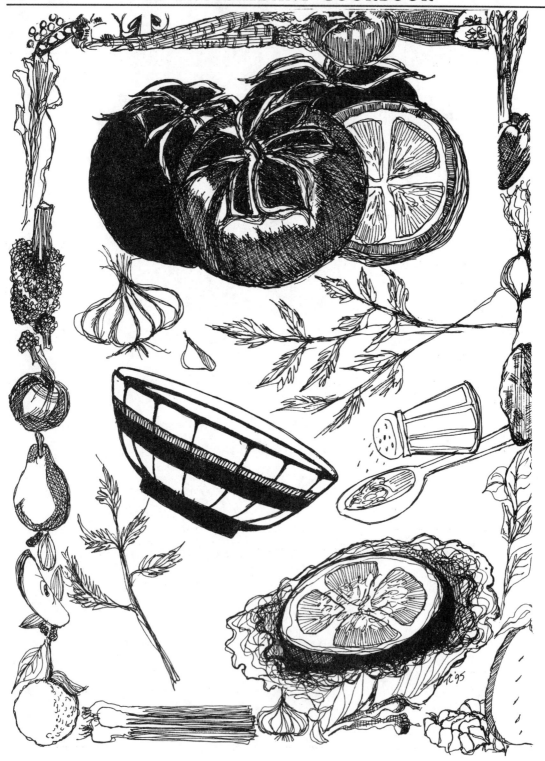

BAKED TOMATOES

1	teaspoon olive oil
4	medium tomatoes
2	teaspoons garlic
5	tablespoons chopped fresh parsley
4	tablespoons bread crumbs
3	tablespoons Parmesan cheese, grated

1. Cut off tops of tomatoes, gently squeeze out seeds, and remove pulpy center to create a hollow for filling.

2. In a small bowl combine garlic, bread crumbs, Parmesan cheese and parsley.

3. Brush oil onto glass baking dish. Set tomatoes into dish. Spoon bread crumb mixture into and onto each tomato.

4. Place in preheated 425 degree oven for 15 minutes or until crumbs are browned.

Rich in the following Antioxidant Nutrients:

Vitamin A	Beta Carotene
Vitamin C	Alpha Carotene
Vitamin E	Lycopene

Plant Antioxidants:

Olive
Oil
Tomatoes
Garlic
Parsley

To enhance antioxidant quotient, add the following: After cooking, add fresh chopped oregano, black pepper, and chopped onion to tomatoes.

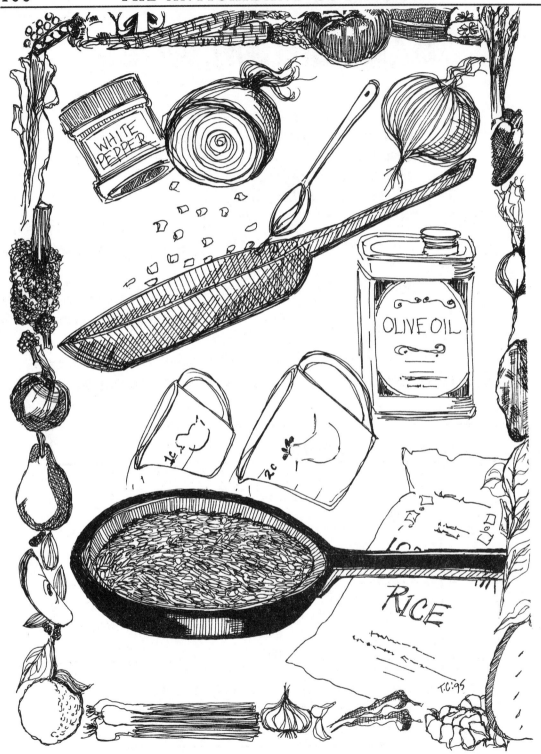

WHITE PEPPER

OLIVE OIL

RICE

T.C.'95

BASIC PILAF

1   tablespoon olive oil
1   medium white onion, finely chopped
1½   cups long grain rice (rinsed until water runs clear)
¼   teaspoon white pepper
3   cups hot chicken broth

1. In heavy (oven ready) saucepan lightly brown onion in the olive oil.

2. Add uncooked rice. Sauté for an additional 5 minutes. Rice should be well coated.

3. Add hot broth. Bring mixture to a boil, stirring constantly. Remove from heat. Cover and put into 325 degree preheated oven for 18 minutes.

Rich in the following Antioxidant Nutrients:

Vitamin A	Beta Carotene
Vitamin C	Alpha Carotene
Vitamin E	Lycopene

Plant Antioxidants:

Olive
Oil
Onion
White Pepper

To enhance antioxidant quotient, add the following: After cooking, add fresh pineapple or papaya and fresh chopped scallions to pilaf.

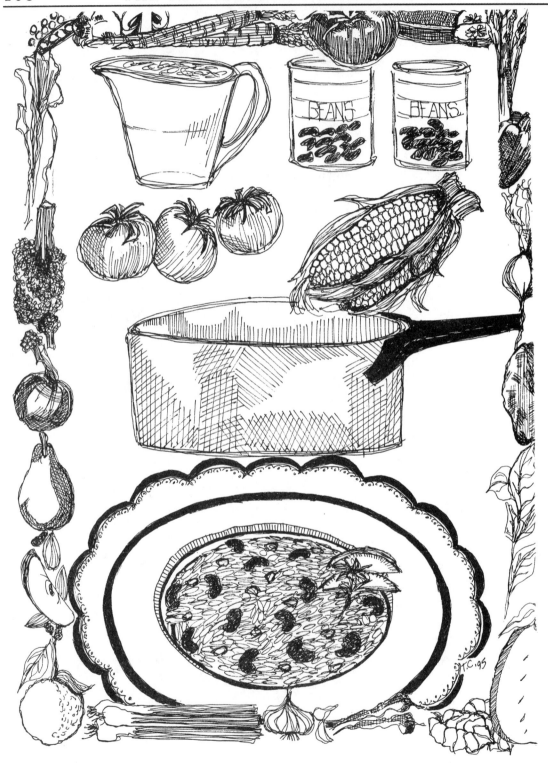

BLACK BEANS & RICE

2   cups, cooked, long grain rice
2   cans (16 ounces) black beans, liquid drained
3   medium tomatoes, chopped
2   ears of corn, cut from the cob and blanched, or substitute
1   10 ounce package frozen whole kernel corn
1   teaspoon cumin
1   teaspoon chili powder
1   medium white onion, chopped
1   teaspoon minced garlic

1. Place all ingredients, except the cooked rice, including the juice from the tomatoes into a medium saucepan. Bring to a boil. Lower heat and simmer for 15 minutes.

2. Spoon over hot rice.

Rich in the following Antioxidant Nutrients:

Vitamin A	Beta Carotene
Vitamin C	Alpha Carotene
Vitamin E	Lycopene

Plant Antioxidants:

Black
Beans
Tomatoes
Corn
Cum in
Chili Powder
Onion
Garlic

To enhance antioxidant quotient, add the following: After cooking, add fresh cucumber slices and chili flakes to beans and rice.

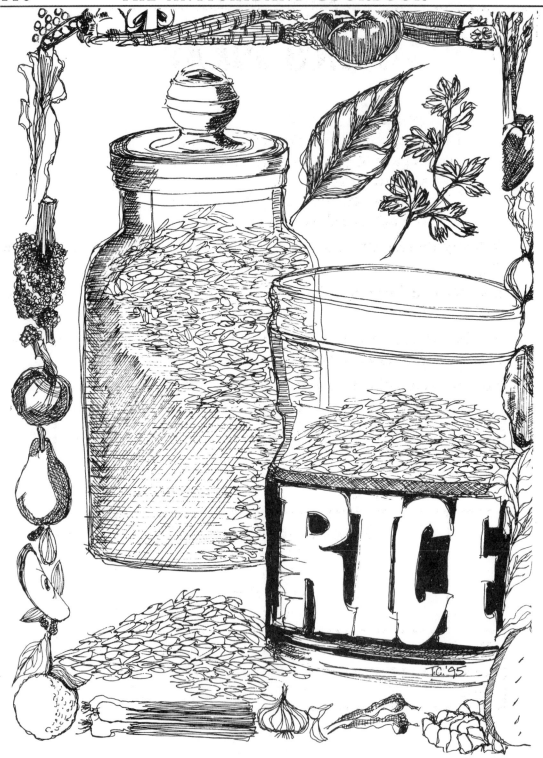

HERB PILAF

1	tablespoon olive oil
1	medium white onion, finely chopped
1½	cups long grain rice (rinsed until water runs clear)
3	cups hot water
2	tablespoons chopped Italian parsley
2	tablespoons chopped basil

1. In heavy (oven ready) deep sauté pan, lightly brown onion in the olive oil.

2. Add uncooked rice. Sauté for an additional 5 minutes. Rice should be well coated.

3. Add hot water. Bring to a boil, stirring constantly. Remove from heat. Cover and put into 325 degree preheated oven for 18 minutes.

4. Fluff rice and sprinkle with fresh herbs.

Rich in the following Antioxidant Nutrients:

Vitamin A	Beta Carotene
Vitamin C	Alpha Carotene
Vitamin E	Lycopene

Plant Antioxidants:
Olive Oil
Onion
Parsley, Italian
Basil

To enhance antioxidant quotient, add the following: After cooking, add chopped white onions, garlic, and pine nuts to pilaf.

JUST SO FRIED RICE

1   white onion, finely chopped
1   tablespoon and 1 teaspoon peanut oil
2   cups white rice, uncooked (rinsed until water is clear)
3   cups chicken broth
2   eggs, slightly beaten
4   scallions (green onions), sliced at a slant
1   handful of bean sprouts
1/4   cup brewed soy sauce
1/4   cup *toasted sesame seeds

1. Sauté onions in 1 tablespoon of peanut oil. Add rice and water and bring to a boil. Cover, lower heat and simmer for 20 minutes.

2. Brush large sauté pan with remaining peanut oil. Heat and add eggs.

3. Stirring constantly, add rice, scallions and soy sauce. Brown lightly. Garnish with bean sprouts and toasted sesame seeds.

*Toasted Sesame Seeds:

Brush a small non-stick sauté pan with a slight amount of oil. Using high heat put in sesame seeds. Stir constantly until seeds are well browned. Approximately 3 minutes.

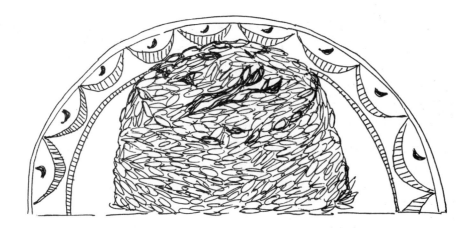

Rich in the following Antioxidant Nutrients:

Vitamin A	Beta Carotene
Vitamin C	Alpha Carotene
Vitamin E	Lycopene

Plant Antioxidants:

Onion
Peanut Oil
Scallions
Bean Sprouts
Soy Sauce
Sesame Seeds

To enhance antioxidant quotient, add the following: After cooking, add fresh shelled raw peas and fresh mandarin orange slices to rice.

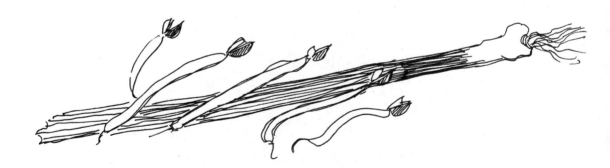

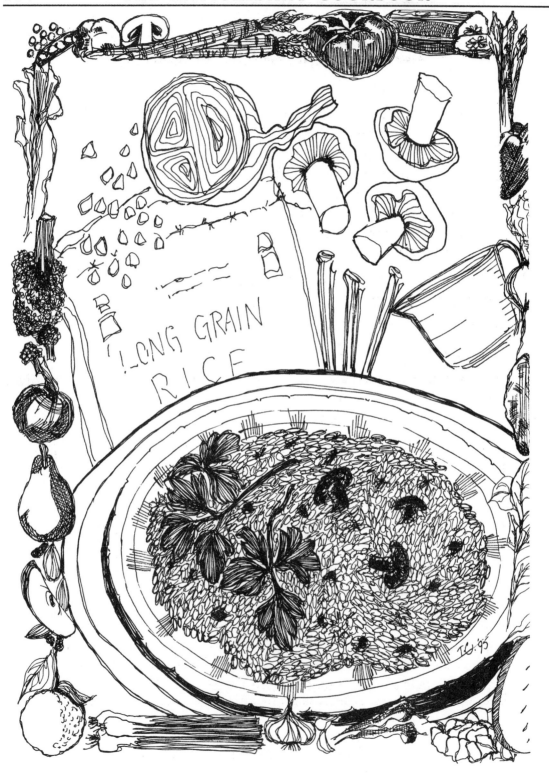

MUSHROOM PILAF

2	tablespoons olive oil
1	large white onion, finely chopped
1/2	pound mushrooms, sliced
1 2/3	cups long grain rice, rinsed until water runs clear
1	teaspoon salt
1/2	teaspoon ground cinnamon
2	cinnamon sticks
3 3/4	cups hot water.

1. Heat oil in large heavy saucepan. Add ground cinnamon and cinnamon sticks. Heat for 2 minutes.

2. Add onions. Sauté until soft.

3. Add mushrooms and sauté for 5 additional minutes.

4. Add rice, sauté for 3 minutes. Add water, bring to a boil. Lower heat, cover and simmer for 20 minutes.

Rich in the following Antioxidant Nutrients:

Vitamin A	Beta Carotene
Vitamin C	Alpha Carotene
Vitamin E	Lycopene

Plant Antioxidants:

Olive Oil
Onion
Mushrooms
Cinnamon

To enhance antioxidant quotient, add the following: After cooking, add cashew pieces and nutmeg to pilaf.

RICE LATINO

(Vegetarian, Tofu, Chicken, Fish, or Turkey)

1½   cups, uncooked long grain rice
2   large white onions, sliced
1   each yellow, and green bell pepper, chopped or diced
¾   pound lean ground beef*
6   medium tomatoes, peeled, seeded, chopped, (3 cups canned
         tomatoes may be substituted here)
2   teaspoons chili paste
½   teaspoon white pepper
½   teaspoon cumin

1. Brown ground beef. Drain most of excess oil from meat.

2. Add in onions and peppers. Cook an additional 2 minutes.

3. Add in tomatoes, chili paste, pepper, cumin and rice. Mix well, bring to
    a boil. Lower heat. Simmer, covered for 20 minutes.

Substitutions: Tofu, Chicken, Fish, or Turkey

Rich in the following Antioxidant Nutrients:

Vitamin A	Beta Carotene
Vitamin C	Alpha Carotene
Vitamin E	Lycopene

Plant Antioxidants:

Onion
Yellow Bell Pepper
Green Bell Pepper
Tomatoes
Chili Paste
White Pepper
Cumin

To enhance antioxidant quotient, add the following: Sliced fresh tomatoes, red peppers, celery and carrots may be added as a garnish.

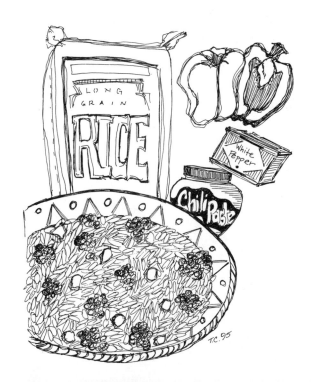

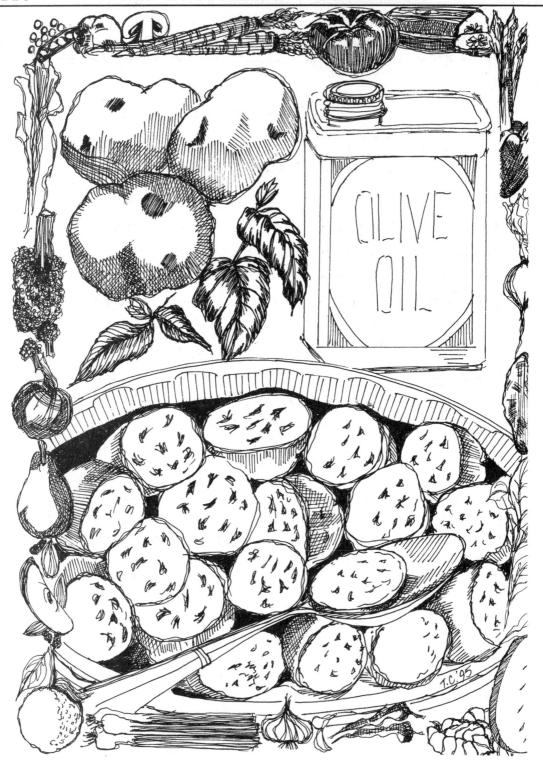

ROASTED RED POTATOES

2   pounds small red potatoes, cut into halves
2   tablespoons olive oil
1/2 teaspoon freshly ground pepper
1   teaspoon chopped (dry) basil

1. Toss potatoes with oil and sprinkle with basil and pepper.

2. In a small roasting pan, arrange potatoes, cut sides down.

3. Preheat oven to 400 degrees, and bake for 20 minutes.

Rich in the following Antioxidant Nutrients:

Vitamin A	Beta Carotene
Vitamin C	Alpha Carotene
Vitamin E	Lycopene

Plant Antioxidants:
Red Skin Potatoes
Olive Oil
Pepper, Black
Basil

To enhance antioxidant quotient, add the following: After cooking, brush white wine vinegar and soy sauce over potatoes, then add fresh chopped garlic to taste.

ROASTED VEGETABLES & RIGATONI

12	ounces rigatoni noodles, cooked al dente, and tossed with 1 tablespoon olive oil and 2 tablespoons chopped dry basil
1/2	teaspoon chili powder (or to taste preference)
1/2	teaspoon paprika (or to taste preference)
3/4	cups olive oil
2	tablespoons apple cider vinegar
1	tablespoon minced garlic
1/4	cup finely chopped shallots
4	Japanese eggplant, each cut into 4 sections
4	yellow squash, cut into 1" slices
1/2	pound mushrooms, halved
2	Bermuda onions, each cut into 8 sections

1. Combine olive oil, apple cider vinegar, shallots, garlic, chili powder and paprika. Coat all vegetables with this mixture.

2. Place vegetables in large glass baking dish; make sure vegetables are not piled up on one another. Bake in preheated 450 degree oven for 15 - 20 minutes.

3. Spoon vegetable mixture over noodles.

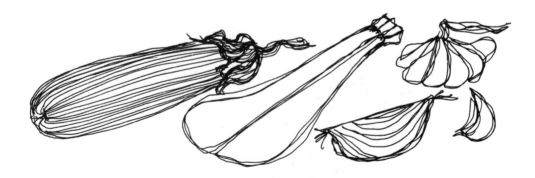

Rich in the following Antioxidant Nutrients:

Vitamin A	Beta Carotene
Vitamin C	Alpha Carotene
Vitamin E	Lycopene

Plant Antioxidants:

Chili Powder
Paprika
Olive Oil
Garlic
Apple Cider Vinegar
Shallots
Eggplant, Japanese
Yellow Squash
Bermuda Onions
Mushrooms

To enhance antioxidant quotient, add the following: After cooking, add strips of fresh red bell pepper and toasted pumpkin seeds to rigatoni.

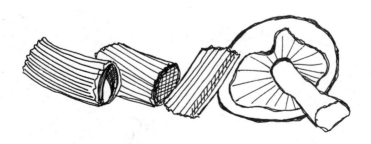

MIXED VEGETABLES

½	large bermuda (red) onion, thinly sliced
½	pound snow peas
1	large red bell pepper, sliced into strips
1	large yellow bell pepper, sliced into strips
½	pound cauliflower, cut into small florets
2	large carrots, julienne
½	pound broccoli florets
1	head butter lettuce

1. Steam broccoli, cauliflower and carrots. Approximately 5 minutes.

2. Spin dry cooked vegetables. Cut into bite-sized pieces. Combine, in a large bowl, with other uncooked vegetables, cut into similar sized pieces. Serve with dressing of your choice. We like the following:

Dressing:

½	cup honey
2	tablespoons walnut oil
1	teaspoon ground orange peel
½	teaspoon ground nutmeg

Combine all ingredients in a small bowl. Mix and drizzle over steamed vegetables. Toss to coat all vegetables. Serve warm.

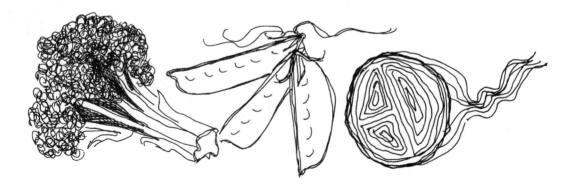

Rich in the following Antioxidant Nutrients:

Vitamin A	Beta Carotene
Vitamin C	Alpha Carotene
Vitamin E	Lycopene

Plant Antioxidants:

Bermuda (Red) Onion
Snow Peas
Red Bell Pepper
Cauliflower
Carrots
Broccoli
Butter Lettuce

To enhance antioxidant quotient, add the following: After cooking, add fresh lemon slices and fresh mango or orange sections to the vegetables.

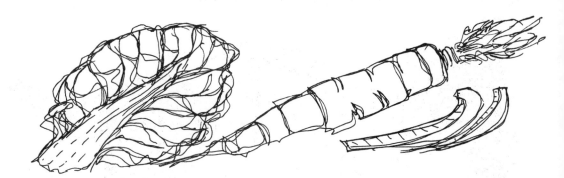

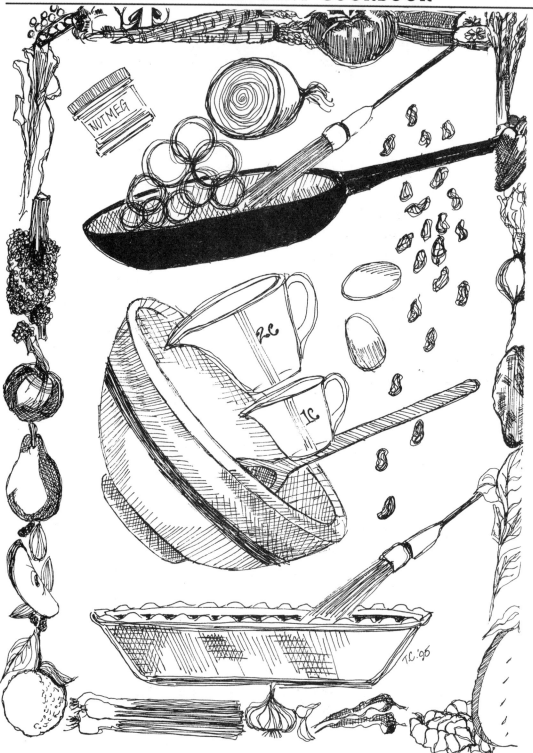

RICE CAKE

2	cups cooked brown rice
1/4	teaspoon nutmeg
2	medium onions, thinly sliced
1/4	cup raisins
2	eggs slightly beaten
4	tablespoons low fat milk
1	tablespoon walnut oil
1	tablespoon water

1. Brush sauté pan and put in onions. Brown the onions, stirring constantly. Add water if needed to help soften onions, as you cook.

2. Combine the onions with rice, eggs, milk and nutmeg in a mixing bowl.

3. Brush glass pie plate with oil.

4. Pour rice mixture into pie plate. Bake at 425 degrees for approximately 20 minutes, or until brown and set.

Rich in the following Antioxidant Nutrients:

Vitamin A	Beta Carotene
Vitamin C	Alpha Carotene
Vitamin E	Lycopene

Plant Antioxidants:

Brown Rice
Nutmeg
Onions
Raisins
Walnut Oil

To enhance antioxidant quotient, add the following: After cooking, add cinnamon powder and sesame seeds to top of the cake.

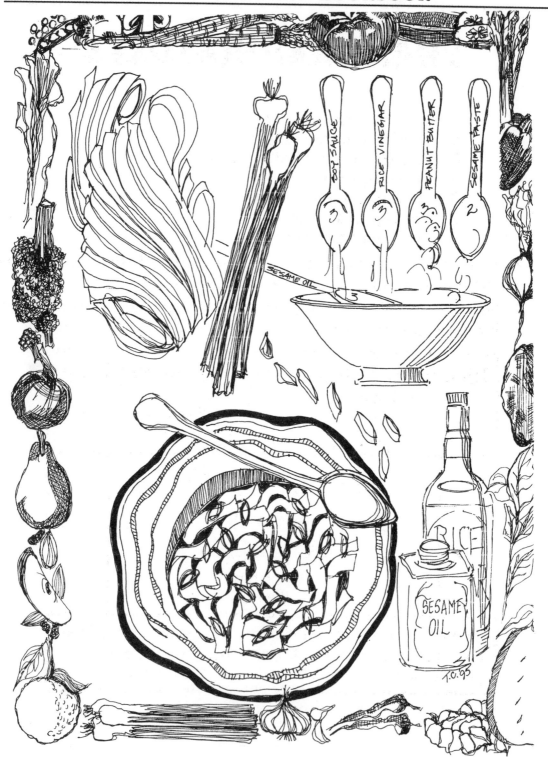

SHANGHAI NOODLES

1	pound egg noodles, cooked al dente
3	scallions, sliced at a slant
3	tablespoons (brewed) soy sauce
3	tablespoons rice vinegar
3	tablespoons peanut butter
2	tablespoons sesame paste
3	tablespoons sesame oil

1. In a medium mixing bowl, mix together peanut butter, sesame paste and sesame oil. Add in soy sauce and vinegar.
2. Place hot noodles in 6 bowls. Spoon equal amounts of sauce over each bowl. Garnish with scallions.

Rich in the following Antioxidant Nutrients:

Vitamin A	Beta Carotene
Vitamin C	Alpha Carotene
Vitamin E	Lycopene

Plant Antioxidants:

Scallions
Soy Sauce
Rice Vinegar
Peanut Butter
Sesame Paste
Sesame Oil

To enhance antioxidant quotient, add the following: After cooking, add fresh shelled raw peas, unsalted ground peanuts, and a few drops of chili oil to the noodles.

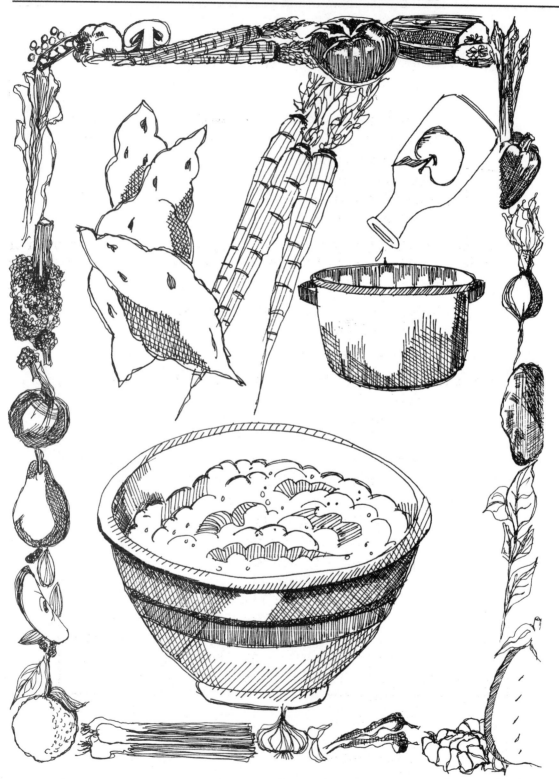

SWEET POTATOES

2½ pounds sweet potatoes, boiled, peeled and chopped
6   medium carrots, scrubbed, chopped and boiled until soft.
⅛   teaspoon ground ginger
¼   teaspoon cinnamon
¼   teaspoon nutmeg
1   quart apple cider

1. Place potatoes and carrots in a large heavy pot such as a Dutch oven or cast iron cooking pot. Add apple cider and enough water to cover vegetables. Bring to a boil, lower heat and simmer until soft.

2. Drain well and put into a bowl. Mash and season with ginger, cinnamon and nutmeg.

Rich in the following Antioxidant Nutrients:

Vitamin A	Beta Carotene
Vitamin C	Alpha Carotene
Vitamin E	Lycopene

Plant Antioxidants:

Sweet Potatoes
Carrots
Ginger
Cinnamon
Nutmeg
Apple Cider

To enhance antioxidant quotient, add the following: After mashing, add pecan pieces, fresh chopped lettuce, and dried raisins or currants to the top of the dish, as a garnish.

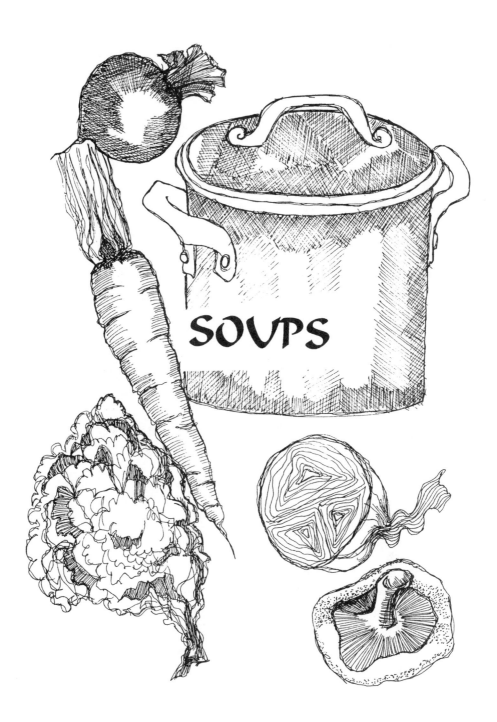

SOUPS

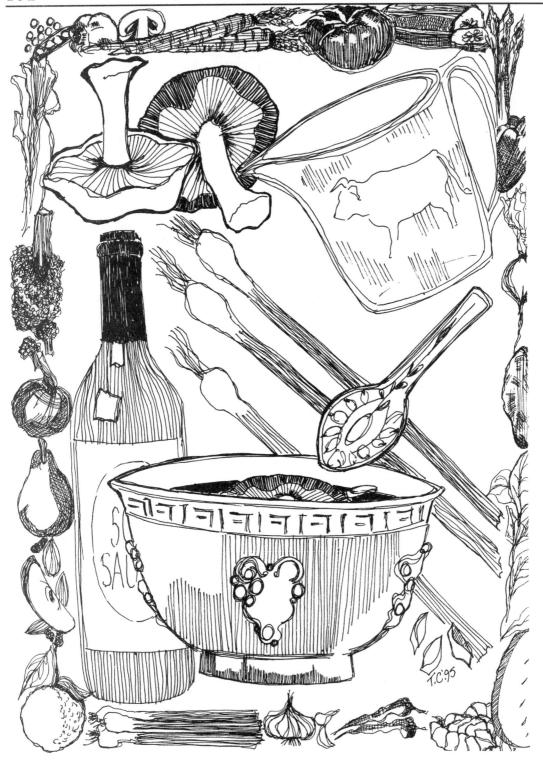

T.C.'95

AU JU SOUP

1   quart beef broth
¼   cup brewed soy sauce
¼   pound shiitake mushrooms, sliced
2   scallions (green onions) the white parts, thinly sliced

1. Heat broth, soy sauce and mushrooms to a boil. Add scallions right before serving.

Rich in the following Antioxidant Nutrients:

Vitamin A	Beta Carotene
Vitamin C	Alpha Carotene
Vitamin E	Lycopene

Plant Antioxidants:
Soy Sauce
Shiitake Mushrooms
Scallions

To enhance antioxidant quotient, add the following: After cooking, add fresh grated ginger to taste.

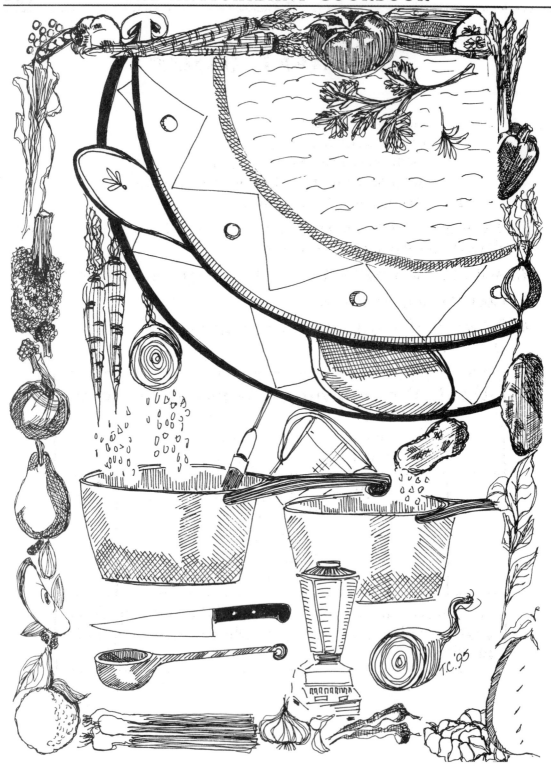

CARROT SOUP

2 teaspoons walnut oil
1 pound carrots, small dice
1 medium white onion, small dice
1 quart and 1 pint chicken or vegetable stock
1 medium potato, small dice

1. Brush inside of heavy saucepan with oil. Add carrots and onions, simmer, covered, until half cooked.

2. Add stock and potatoes. Simmer until all vegetables are tender.

3. Cool, and puree in blender.

4. Reheat soup for serving. If soup seems too thick add additional stock to thin out.

Rich in the following Antioxidant Nutrients:

Vitamin A	Beta Carotene
Vitamin C	Alpha Carotene
Vitamin E	Lycopene

Plant Antioxidants:

Walnut Oil
Carrots
White Onion
Potato

To enhance antioxidant quotient, add the following: After cooking, add crumbled tarragon, white pepper, and ground nutmeg to taste.

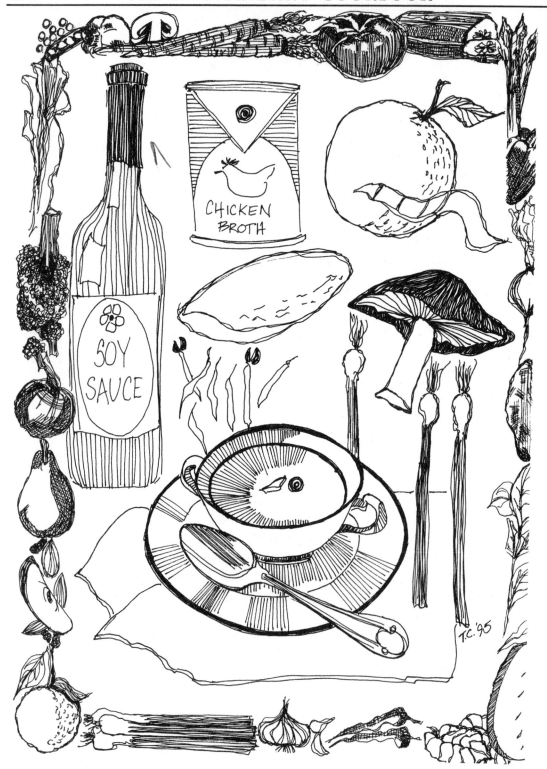

CHICKEN BROTH

SOY SAUCE

T.C. '95

CHINA BROTH

½   cup cooked chicken, julienne
1   handful of bean sprouts
2   teaspoons brewed soy sauce
1   quart chicken broth
1   teaspoon orange peel
5   shiitake mushrooms, sliced
2   scallions (green onions) thinly sliced (use whole onion)

1. Heat broth, soy sauce, and mushrooms to a boil.
2. Add chicken, bean sprouts, orange peel and scallions before serving.

Rich in the following Antioxidant Nutrients:

Vitamin A	Beta Carotene
Vitamin C	Alpha Carotene
Vitamin E	Lycopene

Plant Antioxidants:

Bean Sprouts
Soy Sauce
Orange Peel (Citrus Limonene)
Shiitake Mushrooms
Scallions or Onion

To enhance antioxidant quotient, add the following: After cooking, add fresh chopped lemongrass and fresh grated ginger to taste.

MINESTRONE SOUP

1	tablespoon olive oil
1	medium white onion, thinly sliced
1	medium carrot, small dice
1	teaspoon minced garlic
1	medium zucchini, medium dice
4	large tomatoes, peeled, chopped and pureed
1	quart and 1 pint chicken or vegetable stock
1/4	teaspoon basil
2	ounces elbow or shell macaroni
1	can white beans, drained
	grated parmesan cheese to garnish

1. Heat oil in heavy saucepan. Add onion, carrot and garlic. Cover and cook until softened.

2. Add zucchini, simmer 5 more minutes.

3. Add tomatoes, stock, basil and pasta. Cook until pasta is done.

4. Add beans and bring sauce to a boil.

5. Remove from heat. Season with salt and pepper to taste. Garnish with parmesan cheese.

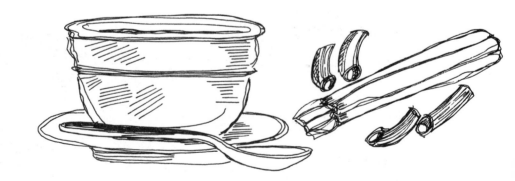

Rich in the following Antioxidant Nutrients:

Vitamin A	Beta Carotene
Vitamin C	Alpha Carotene
Vitamin E	Lycopene

Plant Antioxidants:

Olive Oil
Onion
Carrot
Garlic
Zucchini
Tomatoes
Basil
White Beans

To enhance antioxidant quotient, add the following: After cooking, add fresh chopped parsley and fresh chopped oregano to taste.

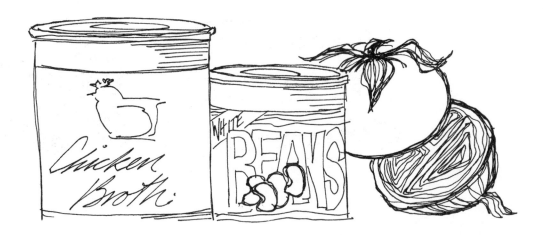

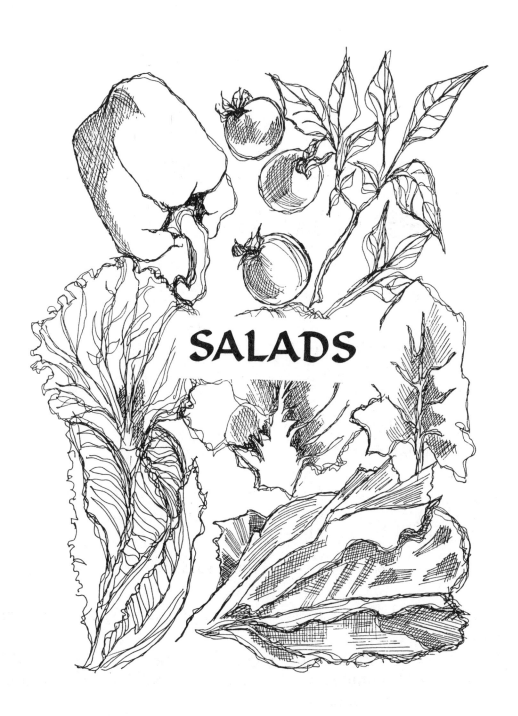

SALADS

ASIA SALAD

1/2	pound linguini, cooked al dente, drained set aside
1	scallion, sliced at a slant
1	medium carrot, scraped and shredded
3	tablespoons (brewed) soy sauce
2	teaspoons sesame oil
1	teaspoon minced garlic
1/2	teaspoon chili flakes
1	teaspoon lemon juice
1	teaspoon lemon peel
2	teaspoons water
	toasted sesame seeds to garnish

1. Combine soy sauce, sesame oil, water, garlic, chili flakes, lemon juice and lemon peel in a small bowl.

2. Combine cooked linguini, soy sauce mixture, carrots, and scallions.

3. Chill. Sprinkle with sesame seeds.

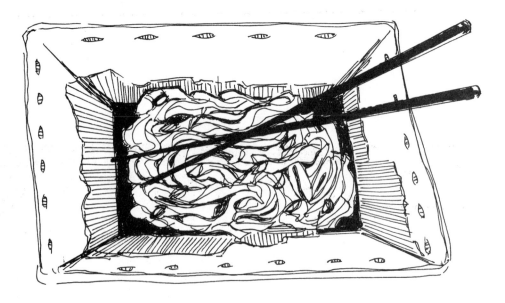

Rich in the following Antioxidant Nutrients:

Vitamin A   Beta Carotene
Vitamin C   Alpha Carotene
Vitamin E   Lycopene

Plant Antioxidants:

Scallion
Carrot
Soy Sauce
Sesame Oil
Garlic
Chili Flakes
Lemon Juice (Citrus Limonene)
Lemon Peel (Citrus Limonene)
Sesame Seeds

To enhance antioxidant quotient, add the following: After preparing, add fresh mint leaves and fresh grated ginger to salad.

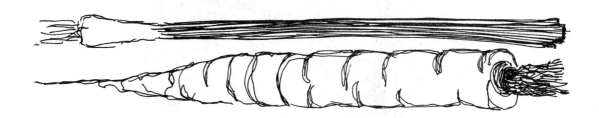

BLACK BEAN SALAD

1	ear yellow corn (removed from cob, and blanched). 1 8 ounce can whole kernel corn can be substituted here.
1	can (16 ounces) black beans, liquid drained
1	red bell pepper, halved, seeded and diced
3	scallions, sliced at a slant
1	medium white onion, chopped
1	teaspoon minced garlic
2	tablespoons fresh cilantro, chopped
	juice of 2 limes
1	teaspoon lime peel
½	cup apple cider vinegar
½	teaspoon chili oil
	salt and pepper to taste

1. Mix all ingredients in large bowl. Allow to marinate an hour or so. Adjust seasonings salt, pepper and chili oil to taste be serving.

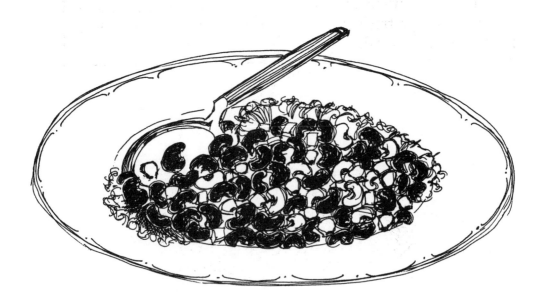

Rich in the following Antioxidant Nutrients:

Vitamin A	Beta Carotene
Vitamin C	Alpha Carotene
Vitamin E	Lycopene

Plant Antioxidants:

Corn
Black Beans
Red Bell Pepper
Scallions
Onion
Garlic
Cilantro
Pepper
Lime (Citrus Limonene)
Apple Cider Vinegar
Chili Oil

To enhance antioxidant quotient, add the following: After preparing, add fresh tomato slices and fresh strips of yellow bell pepper to salad.

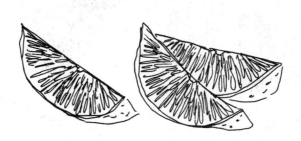

BEAN SALAD

4	cups white beans, cooked
1/4	cup (extra virgin) olive oil
1/2	cup white vinegar
1/4	cup red wine vinegar
4	medium tomatoes, peeled and chopped
2	medium white onions, halved and finely sliced
1	red and 1 green bell pepper, diced
1/2	cup chopped parsley
1/2	pound white albacore tuna (steamed or grilled). (1 6 ounce can of solid, water packed tuna may be substituted for fresh tuna)

1. Combine peppers, parsley and onions.

2. Combine tuna and tomatoes

3. Combine both mixtures, add in beans, vinegars and olive oil. Season with salt and pepper to taste.

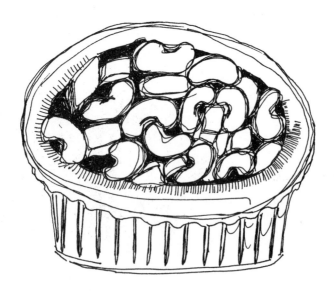

Rich in the following Antioxidant Nutrients:

Vitamin A   Beta Carotene
Vitamin C   Alpha Carotene
Vitamin E   Lycopene

Plant Antioxidants:

White Beans
Olive Oil
White Vinegar
Red Wine Vinegar
Tomatoes
Onions
Green Bell Pepper
Parsley

To enhance antioxidant quotient, add the following: After preparing, add fresh lemon wedges, fresh celery slices, and fresh ground black pepper to salad.

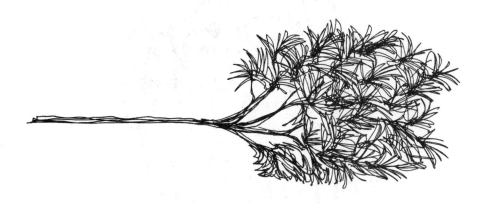

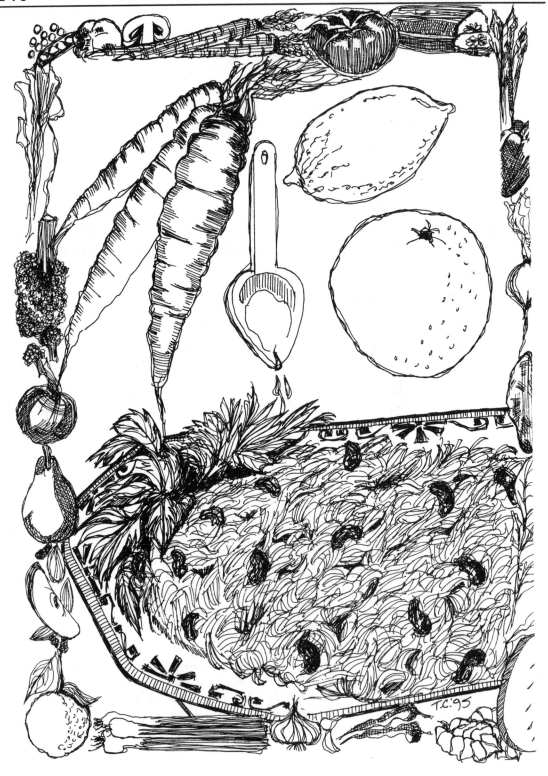

CARROT SALAD

1	pound coarsely grated carrots
2	tablespoons fresh lemon juice
1	tablespoon honey
½	cup raisins
½	cup fresh orange juice
1	tablespoon orange peel

1. In a small sauce pan combine orange juice and raisins. Bring to a boil, lower heat and simmer until raisins are plump. Add additional liquid if needed.

2. Combine lemon juice and honey.

3. Combine carrots, lemon and honey mixture, orange peel and raisins. Mix together well. Chill 30 minutes. Serve cold.

Rich in the following Antioxidant Nutrients:

Vitamin A	Beta Carotene
Vitamin C	Alpha Carotene
Vitamin E	Lycopene

Plant Antioxidants:

Carrots
Lemon Juice
Raisins
Orange Juice (Citrus Limonene)

To enhance antioxidant quotient, add the following: After preparing, garnish with a cup of plain low-fat yogurt and mint sprigs.

CHICKEN SALAD I

Chicken:

4	whole boneless, skinless chicken breasts
1½	red bell peppers, julienne
1	red onion, julienne
1	teaspoon minced fresh ginger
1	tablespoon finely chopped cilantro
1	teaspoon minced garlic
1	teaspoon walnut oil

(For salad bed you will need large red lettuce leaves)

1. Combine cilantro, garlic and oil into a paste. Rub chicken with paste, let stand for 1 hour.

2. Sauté for 15 minutes each side in non-stick pan, cool.

3. Cut chicken into 1½" pieces

4. Combine chicken, red bell peppers, onion and ginger in a bowl.

Dressing:

8	ounces plain yogurt
2	teaspoons cilantro, finely chopped
¾	teaspoon chili flakes
¾	teaspoon (dry) dijon mustard

1. Blend into a liquid.

2. Add dressing to chicken and toss. Let stand for 30 minutes. Spoon salad onto lettuce leaves.

Rich in the following Antioxidant Nutrients:

Vitamin A	Beta Carotene
Vitamin C	Alpha Carotene
Vitamin E	Lycopene

Plant Antioxidants:

Red Bell Peppers
Onion
Ginger
Cilantro
Garlic
Walnut Oil
Dijon Mustard

To enhance antioxidant quotient, add the following: After preparing, add chopped walnuts and chopped pimentos to salad.

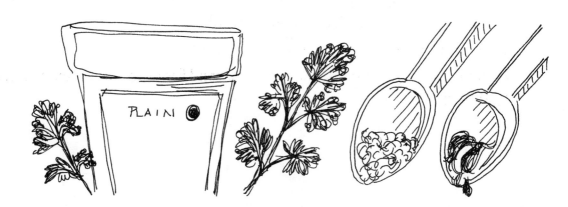

CHICKEN SALAD II

3   cups cooked chicken, shredded.
1   tablespoon sesame oil
1/4   cup seasoned rice vinegar
2   tablespoons soy sauce (brewed variety)
1   teaspoon fresh lemon juice
8   cups finely sliced iceberg lettuce
3   tangelos, or honey tangerines (seedless) peeled and sectioned
        (1 can mandarin oranges 6 ounces drained, may be
        substituted)
3/4   cup sliced (diagonally cut) scallions
3/4   cup fresh cilantro leaves (whole)
1/2   cup sliced water chestnuts
1/4   cup sesame seeds, toasted
6 - 8 large iceberg lettuce leaves

1. Combine vinegar, oil, soy sauce, lemon juice and chicken.

2. Add shredded lettuce, onions, water chestnuts and cilantro leaves, 2/3 of tangerine or mandarin oranges. Toss lightly.

3. Spoon salad onto lettuce leaves. Top with remaining orange slices. Garnish with toasted sesame seeds.

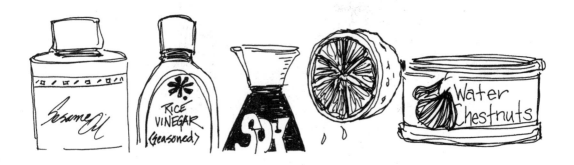

Rich in the following Antioxidant Nutrients:

Vitamin A   Beta Carotene
Vitamin C   Alpha Carotene
Vitamin E   Lycopene

Plant Antioxidants:

Sesame Oil
Rice Vinegar
Soy Sauce
Lemon Juice (Citrus Limonene)
Iceberg Lettuce
Tangelos, Tangerines, or Mandarin Oranges
Scallions
Cilantro
Water Chestnuts
Sesame Seeds

To enhance antioxidant quotient, add the following: After preparing, add fresh chopped cherries or grapes over salad.

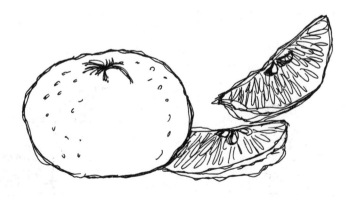

POTATO SALAD I

3	pounds small red potatoes, scrubbed, sliced 1/4" thick
1/2	cup white wine vinegar
2	tablespoons olive oil
1	tablespoon lemon juice
1	tablespoon honey
1	teaspoon oregano
1	tablespoon honey mustard
1/4	cup parsley, coarsely chopped
1	small Bermuda (red onion), finely chopped
1	medium red bell pepper, chopped
4	Italian (turkey) sausages, cooled and cut into 1/2" slices.
3	ounces sundried tomatoes, chopped
	Salt and pepper to taste

1. Boil potatoes 15 – 20 minutes, just until tender. Drain well in colander.

2. Whisk together vinegar, oil, lemon juice and honey mustard.

3. Turn potatoes into a large plastic bag. Add onion, sausage, peppers, tomatoes and dressing. Set bag aside. Let sit for 20 minutes. Turn bag occasionally to distribute ingredients evenly.

4. Serve, slightly warmed, or at room temperature.

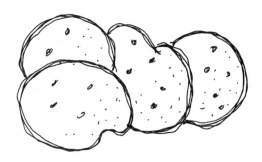

Rich in the following Antioxidant Nutrients:

Vitamin A	Beta Carotene
Vitamin C	Alpha Carotene
Vitamin E	Lycopene

Plant Antioxidants:

Red Skin Potatoes
White Wine Vinegar
Olive Oils
Lemon Juice (Citrus Limonene)
Pepper
Sundried Tomatoes
Oregano
Mustard
Parsley
Red Onion (Bermuda)
Red Bell Pepper

To enhance antioxidant quotient, add the following: After preparing, add ground black pepper, paprika, and fresh rosemary to taste.

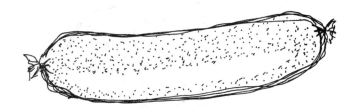

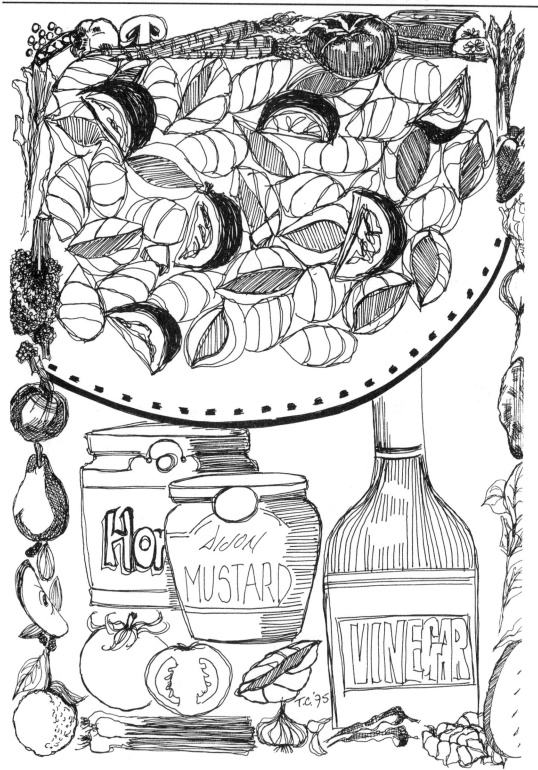

PASTA SALAD

6	ounces pasta shells, cooked, drained, set aside
1	dozen cherry tomatoes, quartered
1	tablespoon honey
1	tablespoon dijon type mustard
2	tablespoons white wine vinegar
4	ounces plain yogurt
1	tablespoon chopped fresh basil
1	cup cooked turkey, cut into 1" pieces

1. Combine pasta, tomatoes and turkey in large bowl.

2. Combine all other ingredients, stir well.

3. Add pasta mixture. Toss to combine all ingredients.

Rich in the following Antioxidant Nutrients:

Vitamin A	Beta Carotene
Vitamin C	Alpha Carotene
Vitamin E	Lycopene

Plant Antioxidants:

Cherry Tomatoes
Dijon Mustard
White Wine Vinegar
Basil

To enhance antioxidant quotient, add the following: After preparing, add fresh raw shelled peas and powdered turmeric to taste.

POTATO SALAD II

3	pounds red potatoes, scrubbed, cut in half and then into wedges
1/2	large red onion, thinly sliced
3	scallions (green onions), thinly sliced
1	tablespoon fresh flatleaf parsley, chopped
1/2	cup plain yogurt
1/2	cup light mayonnaise
1	tablespoon dijon type mustard
1/2	cucumber, peeled, seeded and finely chopped
3	hard boiled eggs, chopped

1. Hard boil eggs, set aside.

2. Boil 4 quarts water, add potatoes, return to boiling. Boil for 15 - 20 minutes, until just tender. Drain well in colander.

3. Mix yogurt, mayonnaise, mustard and cucumber in a small bowl.

4. Turn potatoes into a large bowl. Add yogurt mixture and onions. Mix gently and thoroughly. Add sliced egg. Mix again gently. Garnish with parsley and scallions.

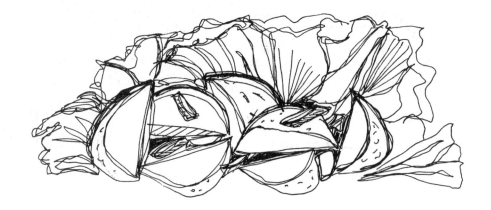

Rich in the following Antioxidant Nutrients:

Vitamin A   Beta Carotene
Vitamin C   Alpha Carotene
Vitamin E   Lycopene

Plant Antioxidants:

Red Skin Potatoes
Red Onion (Bermuda)
Scallions
Parsley, Flatleaf
Dijon Mustard
Cucumber

To enhance antioxidant quotient, add the following: After preparing, add fresh chopped celery and ground cayenne pepper to taste.

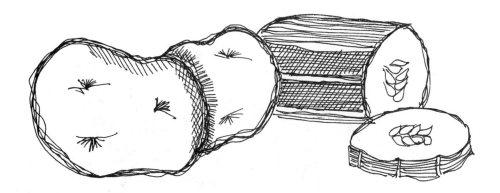

SALSA SALAD

3	scallions, cut at a slant
1	cucumber, peeled, halved lengthwise, seeded, cut into large dice.
1	red bell pepper, large dice
1	large tomato, chopped
1	tablespoon olive oil
2	tablespoons red wine vinegar
1/2	teaspoon chili oil
1	head romaine lettuce

1. Separate white and green parts of onions. Save the green parts, slice the white parts.

2. Combine, in the food processor, the white parts of the onions, red pepper and cucumber. Chop finely.

3. Combine chopped vegetables, tomato, oil, vinegar and chili oil in a small bowl.

4. Arrange lettuce on plates. Spoon the lettuce mixture onto lettuce. Serve cold.

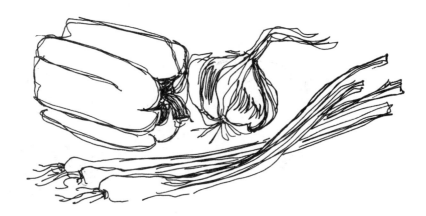

Rich in the following Antioxidant Nutrients:

Vitamin A	Beta Carotene
Vitamin C	Alpha Carotene
Vitamin E	Lycopene

Plant Antioxidants:

Scallions
Cucumber
Red Bell Pepper
Tomato
Olive Oil
Red Wine Vinegar
Chili Oil
Romaine Lettuce

To enhance antioxidant quotient, add the following: After preparing, garnish with fresh lime slices and fresh strips of yellow bell pepper.

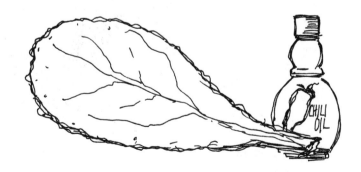

SEAFOOD SALAD

1/8   cup white wine vinegar
1/2   pound medium sized shrimp, shelled and deveined
1/2   pound scallops, cut in halves
1   quart water, with ice in large bowl
1 1/2 teaspoons fresh lemon juice
1 1/2 teaspoons fresh lime juice
1   teaspoon lemon peel
1 1/2 teaspoons dijon type mustard
     *salt for cooking seafood
1/4   cup lite olive oil
1/2   small bermuda onion, minced
1   4 ounce can sliced water chestnuts, drained and chopped
1/2   yellow bell pepper, diced

1. Boil 1 quart salted water (approximately 1/2 teaspoon salt). Add in shrimp. Boil for approximately 1 minute. Remove from water with large strainer, or slotted spoon and put directly into ice water. Do not dispose of cooking water. Allow to set approximately 2 minutes. Drain water. Cut shrimp in halves, lengthwise.

2. Bring water to a boil once again. Add in scallops. Cook 1 to 2 minutes. Drain.

3. Whisk vinegar, lemon juice, mustard, in large bowl. Gently whisk in oil. Add in water chestnuts, bell pepper and onions.

4. Add in scallops and shrimp. Toss to coat. Refrigerate until served.

Rich in the following Antioxidant Nutrients:

Vitamin A	Beta Carotene
Vitamin C	Alpha Carotene
Vitamin E	Lycopene

Plant Antioxidants:

White Wine Vinegar
Lemon (Citrus Limonene)
Lime (Citrus Limonene)
Dijon Mustard
Olive Oil
Red (Bermuda) Onion
Water Chestnuts
Yellow Bell Pepper

To enhance antioxidant quotient, add the following: After cooking, add fresh sliced cucumber and sliced fresh grapes or cherries as a garnish.

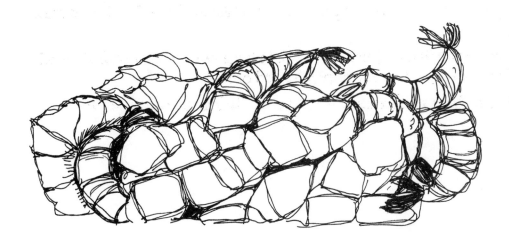

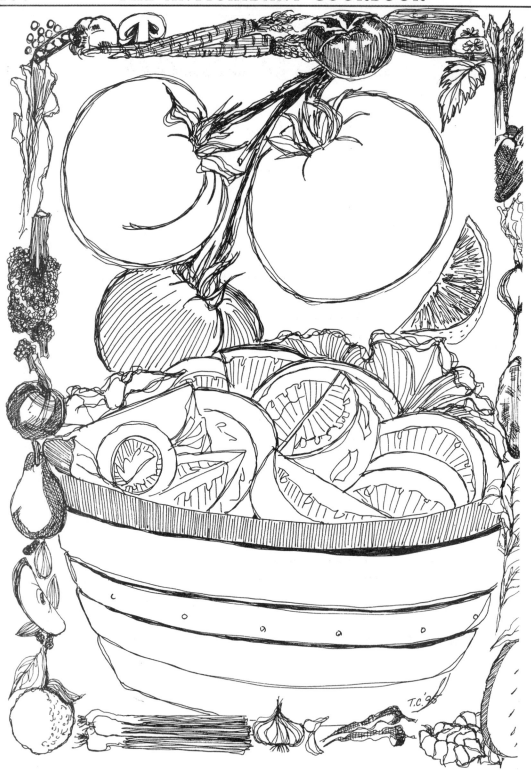

TOMATO SALAD

3   large tomatoes, peeled and chopped
3   scallions, finely chopped
1/4 cup cilantro, chopped
1   tablespoon olive oil
1/2 teaspoon lime juice
1/2 teaspoon lime peel
    salt and pepper to taste

Toss all ingredients. Allow to chill 30 minutes before serving.

Rich in the following Antioxidant Nutrients:

Vitamin A   Beta Carotene
Vitamin C   Alpha Carotene
Vitamin E   Lycopene

Plant Antioxidants:

Tomatoes
Scallions
Cilantro
Olive Oil
Lime (Citrus Limonene)

To enhance antioxidant quotient, add the following: After preparing, add thinly sliced rings of red or yellow onions as well as sliced carrots.

VEGETABLE CHICKEN SALAD

8	ounces low fat yogurt
1	ounce seasoned rice vinegar
1/4	teaspoon white pepper
1	cup cooked chicken breast, cut in 1" cubes
4	cups broccoli flowerettes
1	cup snow peas
1	medium red (bermuda) onion, thinly sliced
2	tablespoons toasted sesame seeds
1/2	cup shredded carrots

1. Combine yogurt, vinegar and pepper in a small bowl, set aside.

2. In a large bowl combine chicken, broccoli, snow peas, onion, sesame seeds and carrots.

3. Toss yogurt dressing with vegetable and chicken. Refrigerate until you are ready to serve this dish.

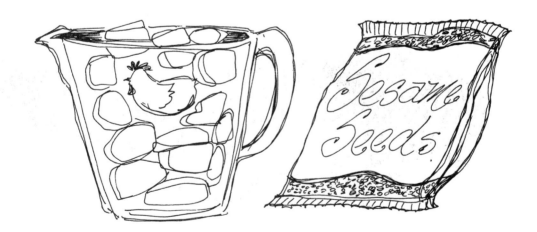

Rich in the following Antioxidant Nutrients:

Vitamin A	Beta Carotene
Vitamin C	Alpha Carotene
Vitamin E	Lycopene

Plant Antioxidants:

Rice Vinegar
Pepper, White
Broccoli
Snow Peas
Red (Bermuda) Onion
Sesame Seeds
Carrots

To enhance antioxidant quotient, add the following: After cooking, add fresh mandarin orange slices and fresh grape halves.

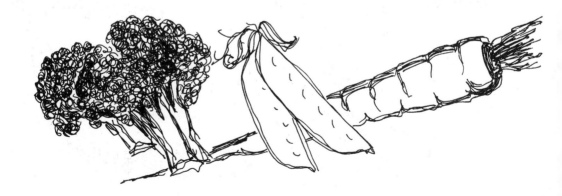

WARM SWEET POTATO SALAD

1	teaspoon walnut oil
2	teaspoons grated and finely chopped fresh ginger
1	green apple, peeled, cored and cut into 1″ pieces
2	pounds sweet potatoes — peeled and cut into 1″ pieces
½	cup golden raisins
1	tablespoon honey
½	teaspoon nutmeg
6	tablespoons grated carrots

1. Brush sauté pan with walnut oil. Over medium heat sauté ginger in pan for 1 minute.

2. Add sweet potatoes, cover, cook stirring occasionally until potatoes are almost tender (approximately 10 minutes).

3. Add apples, raisins, nutmeg and honey, cover and cook at low to medium heat, adding a small amount of water if necessary, an additional 5 to 7 minutes, until potatoes and apples are tender.

4. Garnish with grated carrots.

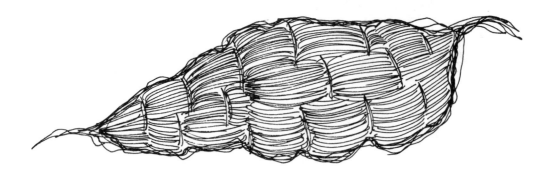

Rich in the following Antioxidant Nutrients:

Vitamin A	Beta Carotene
Vitamin C	Alpha Carotene
Vitamin E	Lycopene

Plant Antioxidants:

Walnut Oil

Ginger

Apple

Sweet Potatoes

Raisins

Nutmeg

Carrots

To enhance antioxidant quotient, add the following: After cooking, add fresh slices of apples and oranges.

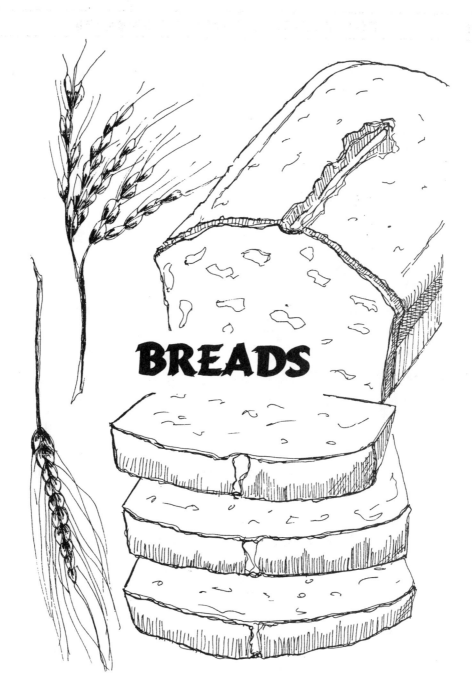

BREADS

POTATO BREAD

2	eggs
1/2	cup honey
3/4	cup cooked, mashed sweet potato
3/4	cup whole wheat flour
1	teaspoon baking powder
1	teaspoon baking soda
1	teaspoon ground cinnamon
1	teaspoon ground ginger
1	teaspoon fresh grated ginger
1	teaspoon vanilla
1	teaspoon safflower oil, to brush coat loaf pan

1. Whisk eggs until foamy.

2. Add mashed sweet potato, honey and vanilla. Whisk for 2 minutes.

3. Combine flour, baking powder, baking soda, cinnamon, ground and grated ginger.

4. Add flour mixture to sweet potato mixture. Mix until all ingredients are well combined.

5. Brush loaf pan with oil. Pour batter into prepared pan. Bake at 375 degrees for 20 minutes or until done. Let cool 5 minutes before removing from pan onto a rack.

Rich in the following Antioxidant Nutrients:

Vitamin A	Beta Carotene
Vitamin C	Alpha Carotene
Vitamin E	Lycopene

Plant Antioxidants:

Sweet Potato
Cinnamon
Ginger
Safflower Oil

To enhance antioxidant quotient, add the following: After cooking, add chopped pecans or walnuts to top of bread.

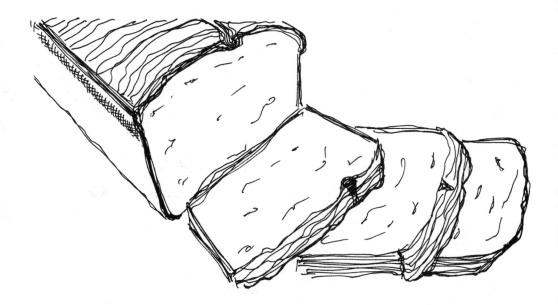

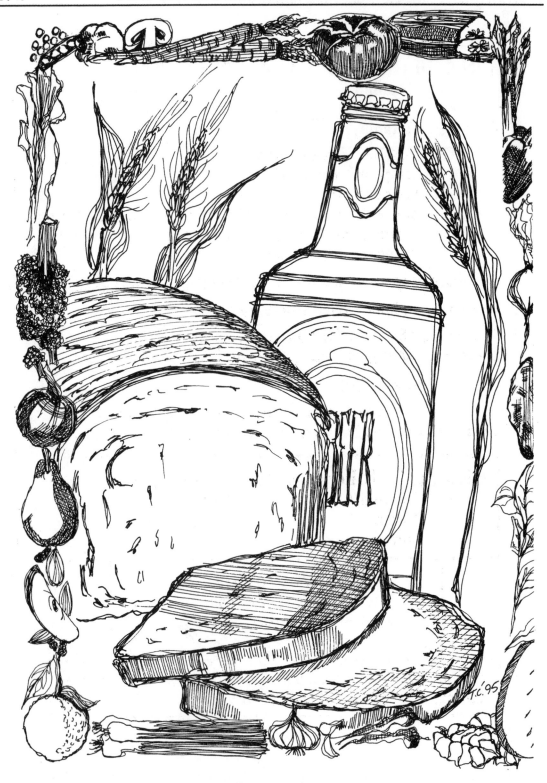

BEER BREAD

2 cups whole wheat flour
¼ cup honey
1 tablespoon baking powder
1 teaspoon baking soda
¼ teaspoon salt
10 ounces beer, (non-alcoholic will do, it's the fermenting process of the beer, not the alcohol, that makes this an important ingredient).

1. In large mixing bowl combine, flour, baking powder, baking soda and salt.

2. Add beer and honey, moisten evenly.

3. Brush a glass 8½" x 4½" loaf pan with safflower or walnut oil. Pour batter into pan. Bake at 400 degrees, until well browned. Approximately 1 hour.

4. Turn onto rack to cool.

For cornbread substitute 1 cup of corn meal for 1 cup of whole wheat flour.
*For softer crust wrap hot bread in parchment, or waxed paper.

Rich in the following Antioxidant Nutrients:

Vitamin A	Beta Carotene
Vitamin C	Alpha Carotene
Vitamin E	Lycopene

Plant Antioxidants:
Whole Wheat Flour
Safflower Oil
Walnut Oil

To enhance antioxidant quotient, add the following: Before baking, sprinkle top of batter with oats.

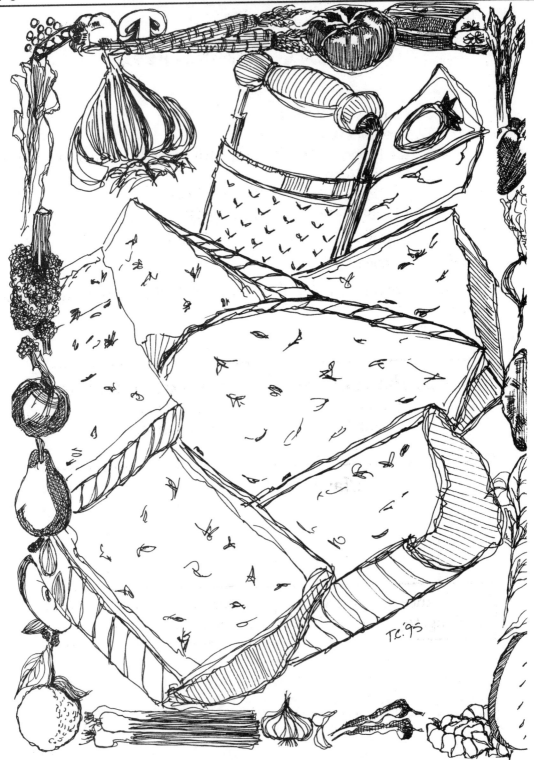

GARLIC BREAD

1 tablespoon olive oil
1 teaspoon minced garlic
1½ teaspoons finely chopped basil or parsley, according to your
own taste
1 tablespoon grated parmesan cheese
½ loaf french bread, cut lengthwise

1. Combine oil, garlic and basil or parsley. Spread onto bread.

2. Sprinkle with cheese.

3. Place under broiler for 1 to 3 minutes. (Watch to insure it does not burn.)

Rich in the following Antioxidant Nutrients:

Vitamin A	Beta Carotene
Vitamin C	Alpha Carotene
Vitamin E	Lycopene

Plant Antioxidants:
Garlic
Basil
Parsley
Olive Oil

To enhance antioxidant quotient, add the following: After cooking, top bread with fresh chopped basil and garlic.

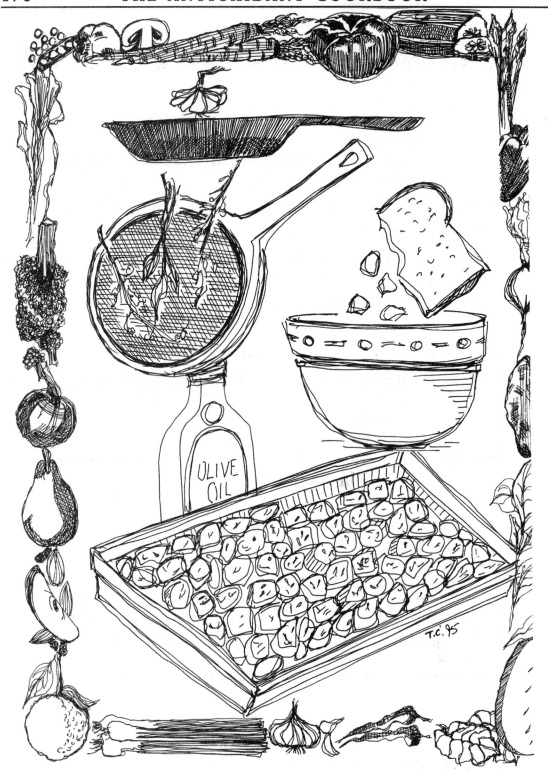

SEASONED BREAD CRUMBS

4 cups whole grain bread, cut into 1" cubes
¼ cup olive oil
½ teaspoon each dry oregano, dry basil and dry thyme
1 tablespoon minced garlic

1. Sauté garlic in oil for 1 minute. Remove from heat. Add herbs.

2. Coat bread cubes with oil/herb mixture.

3. Spread bread onto baking sheet. Bake in preheated 350 degree oven for approximately 7 - 9 minutes, until toasted.

4. Allow to dry thoroughly. Put into food processor to make crumbs.

Rich in the following Antioxidant Nutrients:
Vitamin A	Beta Carotene
Vitamin C	Alpha Carotene
Vitamin E	Lycopene

Plant Antioxidants:
Olive Oil
Oregano
Basil
Thyme
Garlic

To enhance antioxidant quotient, add the following: After cooking, add sesame seeds and chopped fresh parsley to bread crumbs.

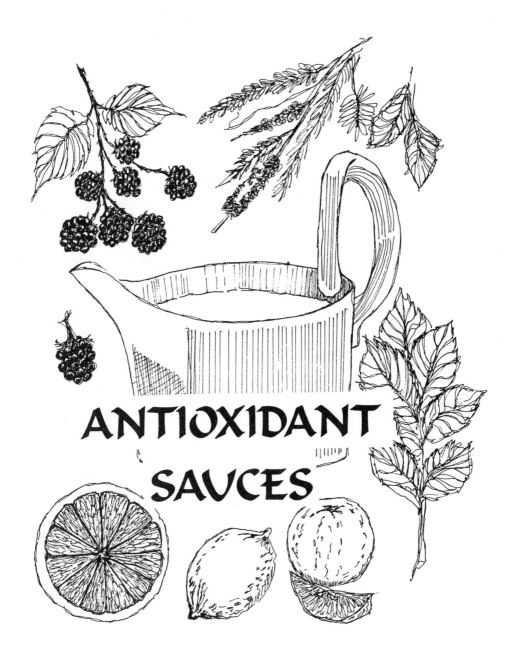

ANTIOXIDANT
SAUCES

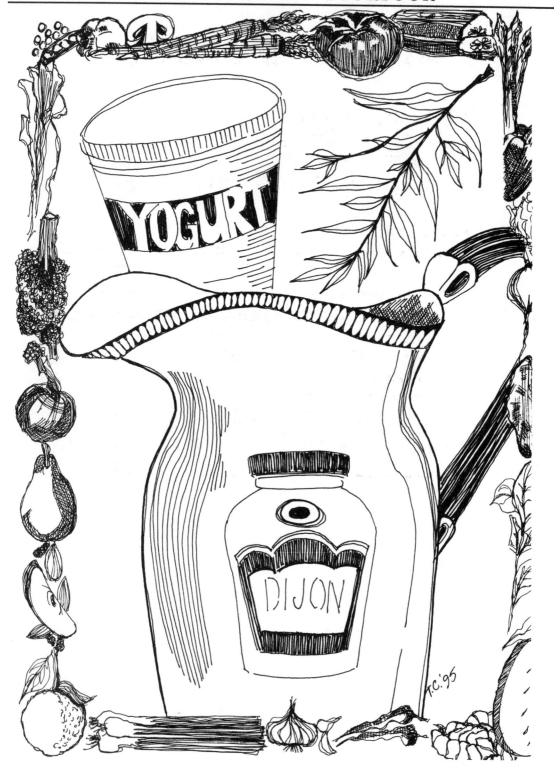

MUSTARD SAUCE

¼   cup Dijon mustard
¾   cup low fat plain yogurt
1½   teaspoon tarragon leaves

1. Combine all ingredients. Blend until slightly thickened.

This is an excellent all-purpose condiment sauce that can be used for chicken, fish and meat dishes as well as on steamed vegetables or rice.

Rich in the following Antioxidant Nutrients:
Vitamin A	Beta Carotene
Vitamin C	Alpha Carotene
Vitamin E	Lycopene

Plant Antioxidants:
Dijon Mustard
Tarragon

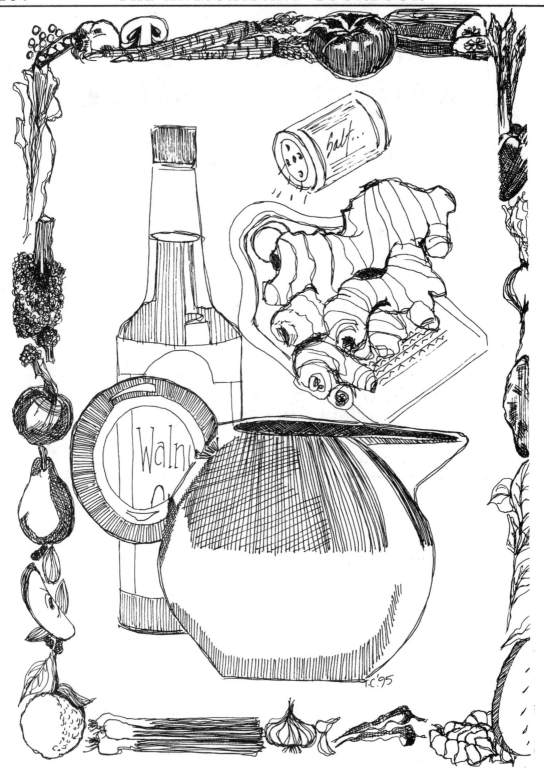

FRESH GINGER ANTIOXIDANT SAUCE

1   fresh whole ginger root (1/2 pound)
1/4 cup walnut oil

1. Peel and scrape ginger root.

2. Shred with cheese grater, then cut and dice.

3. Add walnut oil in mortar.

4. Mash and combine ingredients using mortar and pestle. (If you have a blender, mix very briefly.) Serve at once as a condiment for chicken, fish, and steamed vegetable dishes.

Rich in the following Antioxidant Nutrients:

Vitamin A	Beta Carotene
Vitamin C	Alpha Carotene
Vitamin E	Lycopene

Plant Antioxidants:

Ginger
Walnut Oil

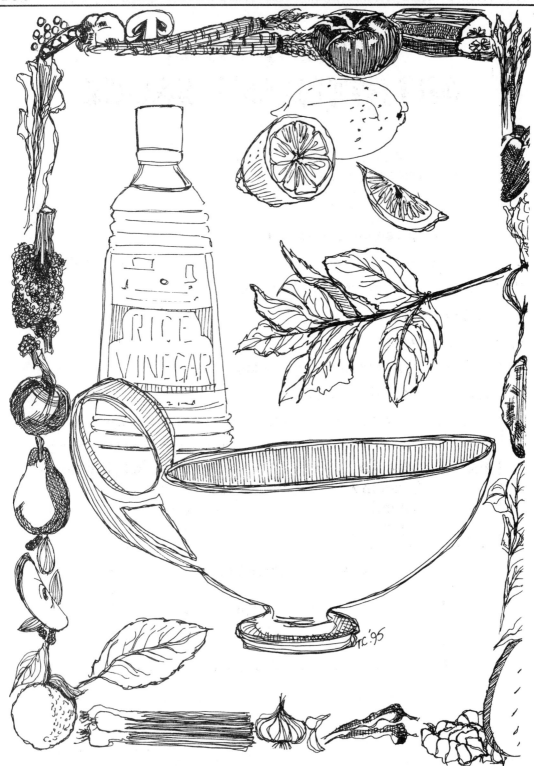

FRESH MINT ANTIOXIDANT SAUCE

1 bunch fresh mint
   juice of one lemon
1 cup rice vinegar
1 whole garlic
   salt and pepper to taste

1. Clean mint in clear running water. Remove all stem material.
2. Chop mint leaves and put in mortar.
3. Add lemon juice.
4. Add rice vinegar.
5. Mash together with pestle in mortar.
6. Season to taste with garlic, salt and pepper.

Add mint sauce as a condiment with meat and chicken dishes.

Rich in the following Antioxidant Nutrients:

Vitamin A	Beta Carotene
Vitamin C	Alpha Carotene
Vitamin E	Lycopene

Plant Antioxidants:

Mint
Lemon (Citrus Limonene)
Garlic
Pepper

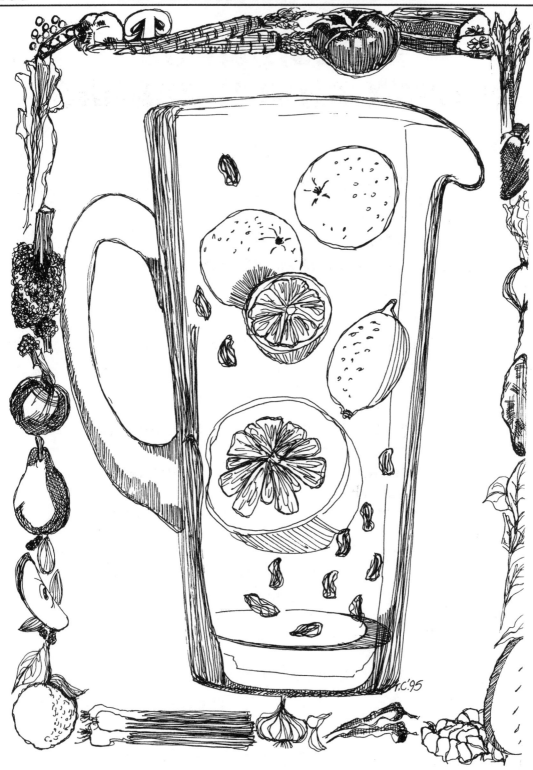

FRESH CITRUS ANTIOXIDANT DRESSING

3	oranges
2	lemons
1	grapefruit
1/4	cup walnut oil
2	ounces golden raisins

1. Extract juice from all fruit, place in blender.

2. Add walnut oil and blend together.

3. Add raisins.

This is a delicious and refreshing summer salad dressing. Added tip: sprinkle nuts on top of salad.

Rich in the following Antioxidant Nutrients:

Vitamin A	Beta Carotene
Vitamin C	Alpha Carotene
Vitamin E	Lycopene

Plant Antioxidants:

Grapefruit, Lemon, & Orange
(Citrus Limonene)
Walnut Oil
Grapes (Raisins, Dried)

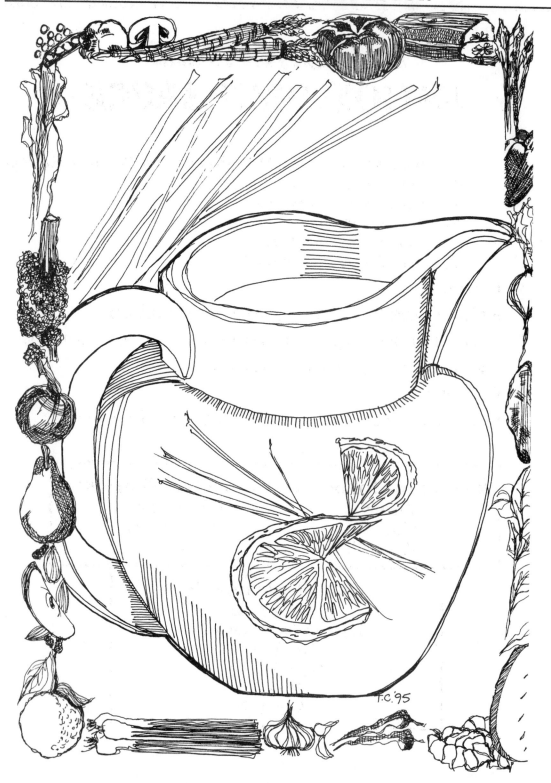

LEMONGRASS ANTIOXIDANT SAUCE

2   ounces fresh lemongrass herb or 6 lemongrass herb tea bags.
8   ounces fresh water
1   ounces lemon juice (fresh)
1/4   cup rice vinegar
1   teaspoon dijon mustard
1/4   cup olive oil or walnut oil

1. Boil water.

2. Add lemongrass herb or tea bags and brew for 5 minutes.

3. Remove herb or tea bags and allow beverage to cool for 10 minutes.

4. Add dijon mustard, rice vinegar, lemon juice and oil.

5. Blend well.

Use as a condiment or dressing for salads and steamed vegetables.

Rich in the following Antioxidant Nutrients:

Vitamin A	Beta Carotene
Vitamin C	Alpha Carotene
Vitamin E	Lycopene

Plant Antioxidants:

Lemongrass
Lemon (Citrus Limonene)
Rice Vinegar
Dijon Mustard
Olive Oil
Walnut Oil

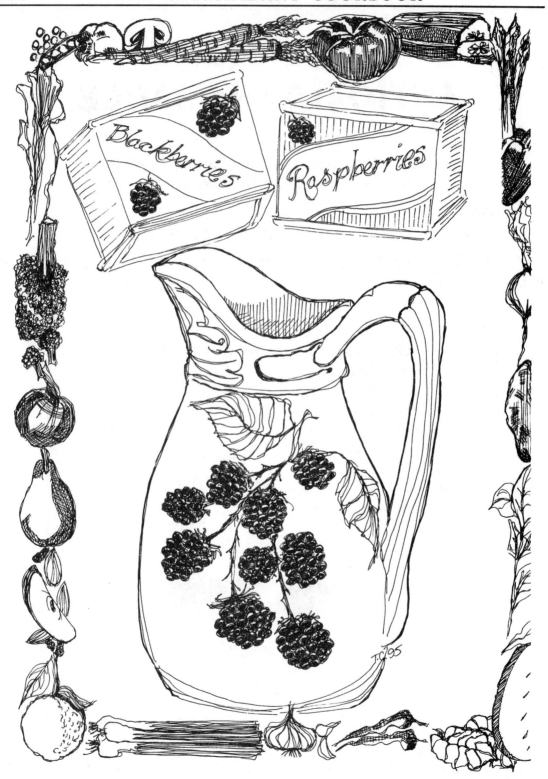

BERRY ANTIOXIDANT SAUCE

1   package frozen raspberries (no sugar added)
1   package frozen blackberries (no sugar added)

1. Defrost according package instructions.

2. Place all berries together in blender. Blend until "smooth."

Cut up fresh fruit of your choice: Bananas, papaya, oranges, kiwi, etc., and pour this antioxidant-rich sauce over the fruit for a superfood taste treat.

Rich in the following Antioxidant Nutrients:

Vitamin A	Beta Carotene
Vitamin C	Alpha Carotene
Vitamin E	Lycopene

Plant Antioxidants:

Raspberries
Blackberries

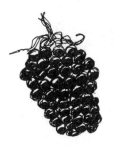

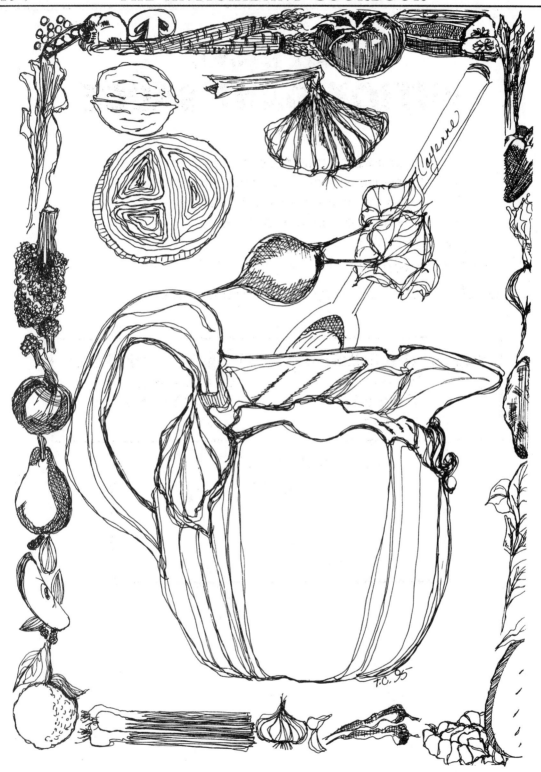

CAYENNE ANTIOXIDANT SAUCE

1   teaspoon cayenne pepper
1   teaspoon ground fresh garlic
1   teaspoon ground fresh white onion
1   teaspoon ground fresh radish
1/3 cup walnut or olive oil

1. Blend all ingredients.

An excellent sauce for shrimp, chicken and fish recipes.

Rich in the following Antioxidant Nutrients:

Vitamin A	Beta Carotene
Vitamin C	Alpha Carotene
Vitamin E	Lycopene

Plant Antioxidants:
Cayenne
Garlic
Onion
Radish
Walnut or Olive Oil

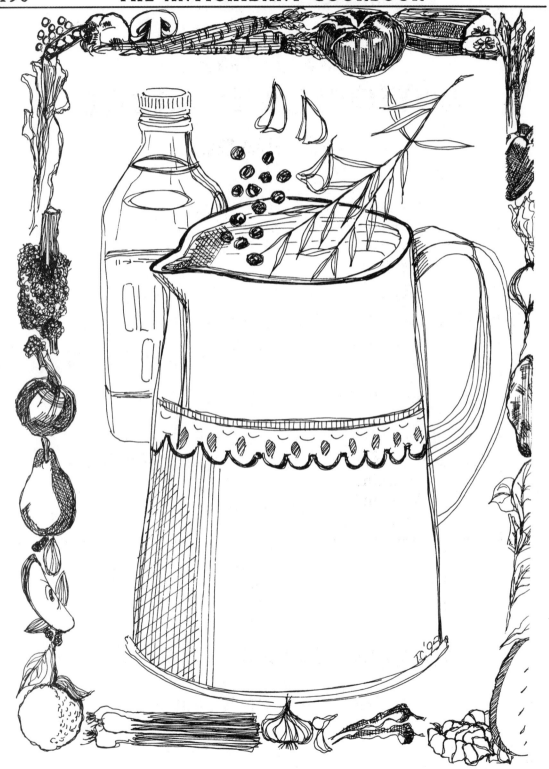

ROSEMARY ANTIOXIDANT SAUCE
(MARINADE)

1   teaspoon rosemary leaves (dried)
1   teaspoon garlic (fresh ground)
1   teaspoon cracked black pepper, ground
1/3   cup olive oil

1. Blend all ingredients.

2. Prepare chicken, fish or meat for broiling. Brush on sauce.

3. Watch broiling process carefully, being sure to keep adding sauce when you turn the food.

This sauce may also be used as a marinade and a condiment.

Rich in the following Antioxidant Nutrients:

Vitamin A	Beta Carotene
Vitamin C	Alpha Carotene
Vitamin E	Lycopene

Plant Antioxidants:
Rosemary
Garlic
Black Pepper
Olive Oil

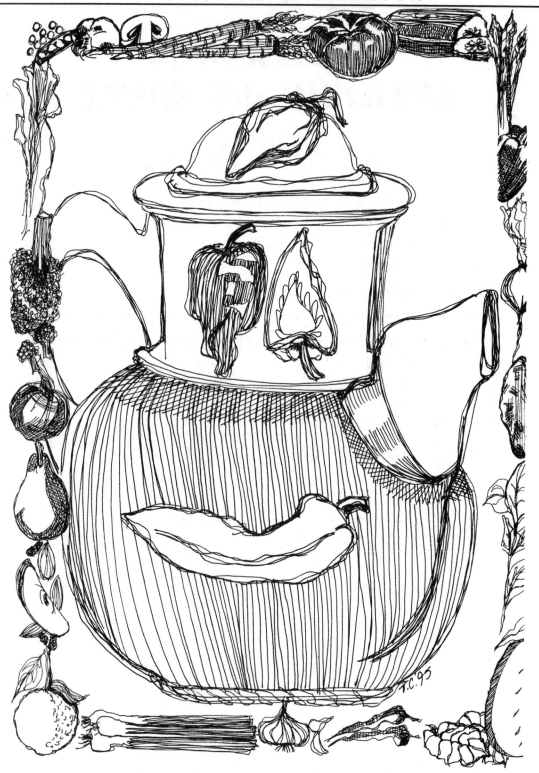

GREEN CHILI ANTIOXIDANT SAUCE

½   teaspoon chopped and diced fresh green chilies (not too spicy hot)
½   teaspoon minced crushed garlic
½   cup white wine vinegar
½   teaspoon warmed honey

1. Blend all ingredients.
2. Chill and reblend just prior to serving.

Rich in the following Antioxidant Nutrients:

Vitamin A	Beta Carotene
Vitamin C	Alpha Carotene
Vitamin E	Lycopene

Plant Antioxidants:

Green Chilies
Garlic
Wine Vinegar

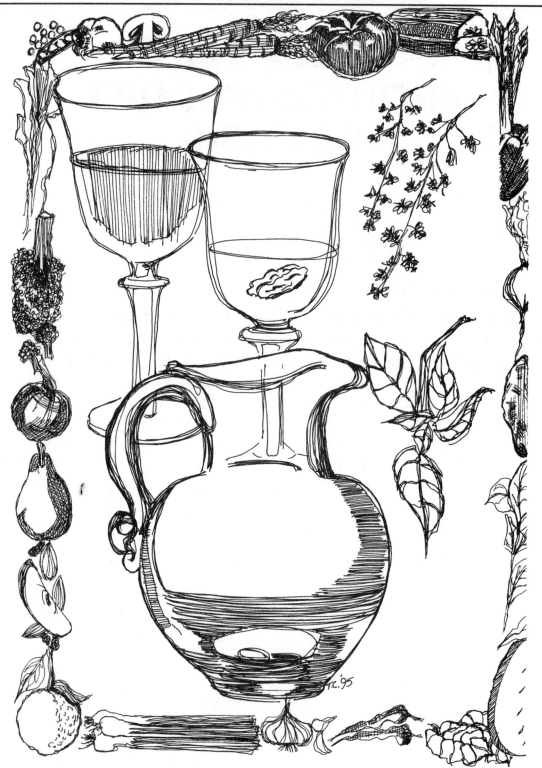

BASIL & OREGANO ANTIOXIDANT SAUCE DRESSING

1   teaspoon oregano (fresh or dried)
1   teaspoon basil (fresh or dried)
1/2 cup red wine vinegar
1/4 cup walnut oil

1. Blend all ingredients for 20-25 seconds at a medium speed, in blender.

Serve over red skin potatoes, raviolis or steamed vegetables.

Rich in the following Antioxidant Nutrients:

Vitamin A	Beta Carotene
Vitamin C	Alpha Carotene
Vitamin E	Lycopene

Plant Antioxidants:
Oregano
Basil
Red Wine Vinegar
Walnut Oil

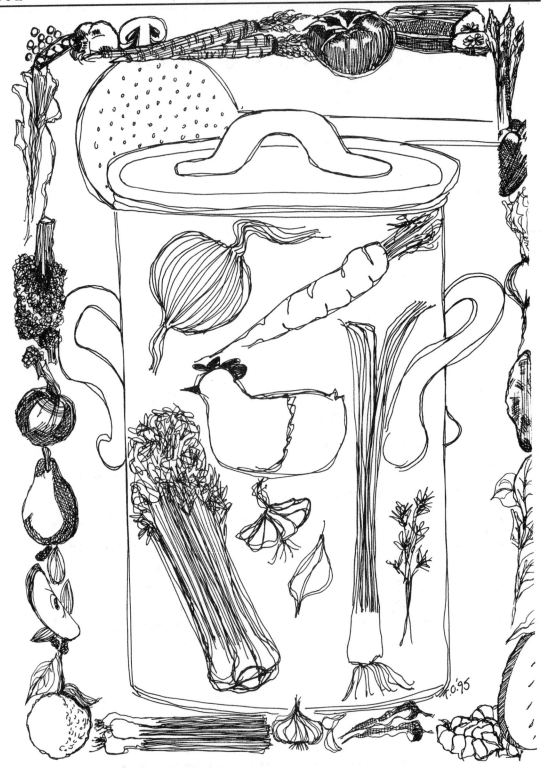

CHICKEN STOCK

6   cups water
1   onion, chopped
1   garlic clove bunch
5   carrots, chopped
2   celery stems, chopped
       sprinkle black pepper, ground

From a whole, quartered fryer, take the parts you normally would not eat:
       the back,
       the "bottom,"
       the giblets,
       the neck.

1. Boil 6 cups of water.

2. Add chicken parts.

3. Add 1 chopped onion, 1 whole chopped garlic clove bunch, 5 chopped carrots,and 2 stems chopped celery

4. Add ground black pepper to taste

5. Simmer for one hour. Strain. Discard solid material, Stock remains.

Makes 4 cups chicken stock.

Rich in the following Antioxidant Nutrients:

Vitamin A	Beta Carotene
Vitamin C	Alpha Carotene
Vitamin E	Lycopene

Plant Antioxidants:

Onion
Garlic
Carrots
Celery
Black Pepper, Ground

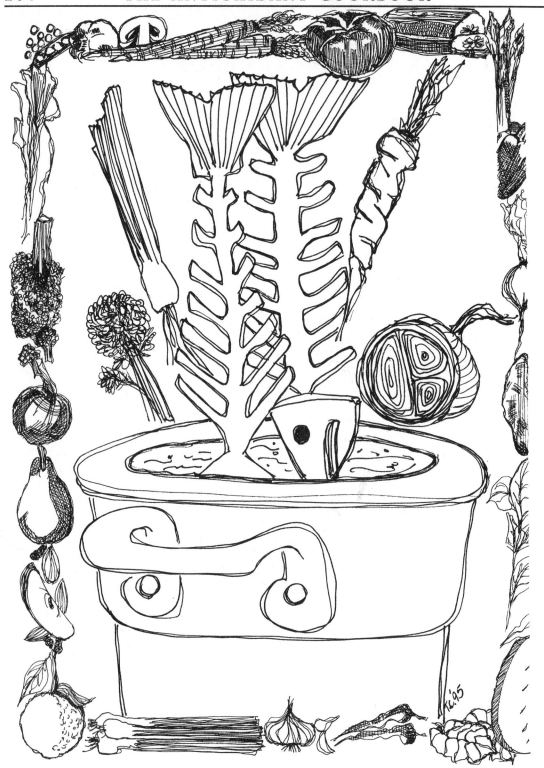

FISH STOCK

4   cups water
1   onion, chopped
1   garlic clove bunch
2   carrots, chopped
1   celery stem, chopped
1   radish, sliced
     sprinkle black pepper or sliced ginger

From a whole fish remove the head, the tail, interior bones, any skin you will not use in cooking the filet fish

1. Bring 4 cups of water to a boil

2. Add fish parts.

3. Add 1 chopped onion, 1 whole chopped garlic clove bunch, 2 chopped carrots, 1 stem chopped celery, and 1 sliced radish.

4. Add ground black pepper or ginger to taste.

5. Simmer for 45 minutes. Strain. Discard solid material, Stock remains.

Makes 3 cups fish stock.

Rich in the following Antioxidant Nutrients:

Vitamin A	Beta Carotene
Vitamin C	Alpha Carotene
Vitamin E	Lycopene

Plant Antioxidants:

Onion
Garlic
Carrots
Celery
Radish
Black Pepper or Ginger

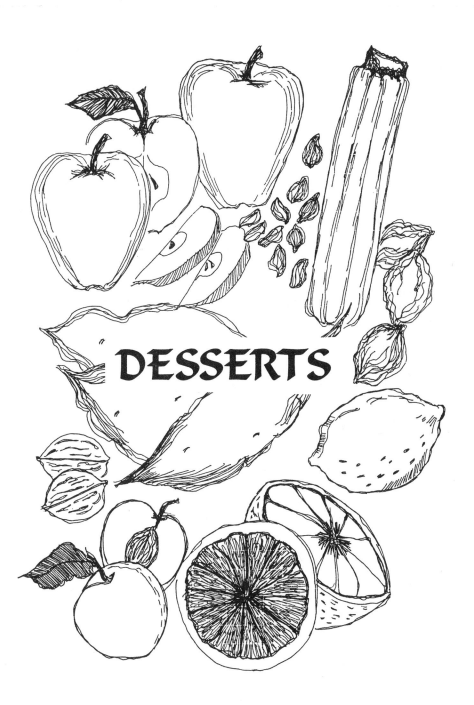

DESSERTS

APPLE TART

Crust:

See recipe for "No Oil Pie Crust" (page 213). Prepare crust and press into medium glass pie plate. Press enough crust to go a little beyond the edge of the pie plate.

Filling:

4	cups cored, grated (shredded) apples
1/4	cup chopped walnuts
1/4	cup golden raisins
1/2	cup honey
1	teaspoon cinnamon
2	tablespoons lemon juice
1	teaspoon ground lemon peel
2	tablespoons cornstarch

1. Combine apples, nuts and raisins in large bowl. Set aside.

2. Combine lemon juice and cornstarch.

3. Combine honey, cinnamon and lemon juice mixture in small saucepan. Bring to a boil, reduce heat and simmer for 1 minute. Pour over apple mixture.

4. Pour mixture into pie plate. Fold over edge of crust. Bake at 350 degrees for 45 minutes.

Rich in the following Antioxidant Nutrients:

Vitamin A	Beta Carotene
Vitamin C	Alpha Carotene
Vitamin E	Lycopene

Plant Antioxidants:
Apples
Walnuts
Raisins
Cinnamon
Lemon (Citrus Limonene)

To enhance antioxidant quotient, add the following: After cooking, top with chopped fresh apples, papaya, berries, or mango.

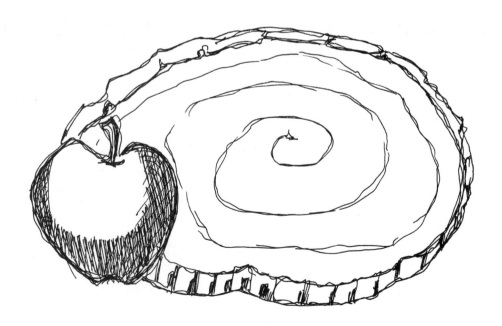

BAKED APPLES

1	teaspoon shredded fresh ginger
5	tablespoons honey
4	tablespoons coarsely ground walnuts
4	tablespoons chopped golden raisins
4	golden delicious apples, cored, top half peeled
	juice of 1 lemon
1	teaspoon lemon peel
1	cup water

1. Combine honey, ginger, walnuts and raisins in a bowl.

2. Rub the peeled tops of the apples with lemon juice.

3. Loosely fill apples with ginger mixture, packing most of the mixture around the unpeeled half of the apple.

4. Place apples in baking dish, Add water to cover the bottom of the dish.

5. Bake at 350 degrees for approximately 1 hour.

6. Put these in the oven as you start preparing dinner. They will be ready to eat as dessert.

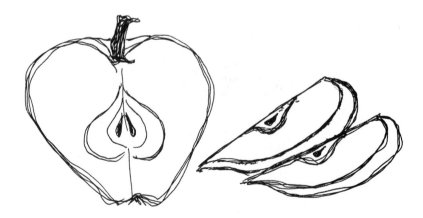

Rich in the following Antioxidant Nutrients:

Vitamin A	Beta Carotene
Vitamin C	Alpha Carotene
Vitamin E	Lycopene

Plant Antioxidants:
Ginger
Walnuts
Raisins
Apples
Lemon (Citrus Limonene)

To enhance antioxidant quotient, add the following: After cooking, top with fresh chopped berries, apples, oranges, or cherries.

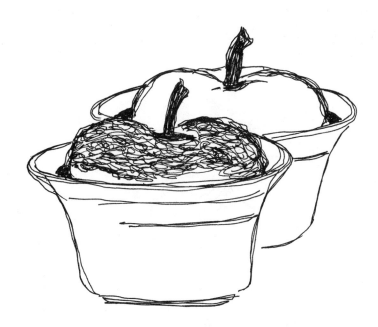

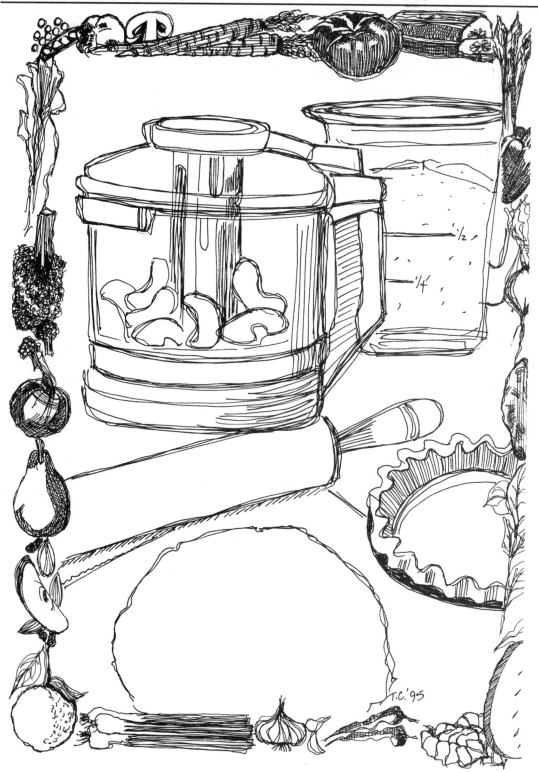

NO OIL PIE CRUST

(This recipe is from Michael Weiner's *Healing Children Naturally*)

1	cup cashews
½	teaspoon salt
½	cup water
1	cup whole wheat flour

1. In a food processor or blender, blend cashews, water and salt until smooth. Remove to a bowl.

2. Add flour to make soft pastry dough.

3. Press into large, shallow, glass pie plate. Bake at 375 degrees for 10 minutes.

Rich in the following Antioxidant Nutrients:

Vitamin A	Beta Carotene
Vitamin C	Alpha Carotene
Vitamin E	Lycopene

Plant Antioxidants:

Cashews

Whole Wheat Flour

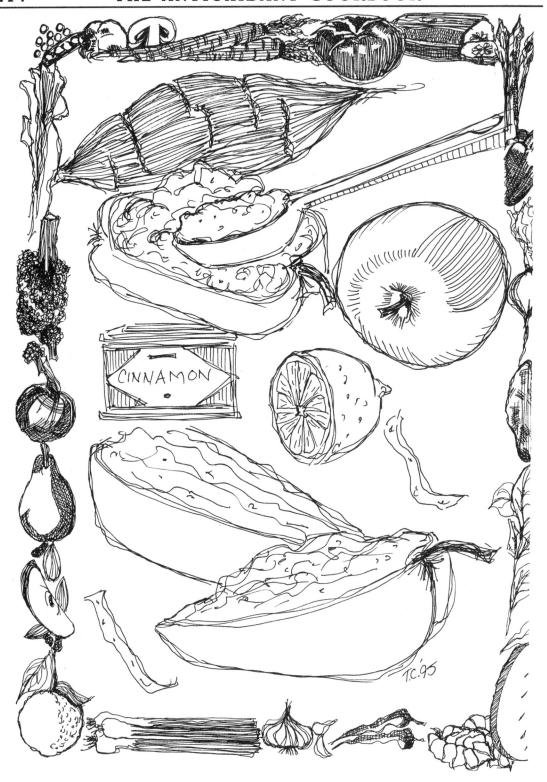

SWEET POTATO CUPS

4	medium sweet potatoes
2	tablespoons honey
4	red delicious apples
1	teaspoon cinnamon
1	teaspoon lemon peel

1. Scrub potatoes, boil until tender, peel and mash.

2. Add honey, cinnamon, and lemon peel to potatoes.

3. Scoop out inside of apples. Chop edible insides and mix with potatoes. Fill apple cups with potato and apple mixture.

4. Bake until apples are cooked (approximately 15 minutes in 325 degree oven).

Rich in the following Antioxidant Nutrients:

Vitamin A	Beta Carotene
Vitamin C	Alpha Carotene
Vitamin E	Lycopene

Plant Antioxidants:

Sweet Potatoes
Apples
Cinnamon
Lemon (Citrus Limonene)

To enhance antioxidant quotient, add the following: After cooking, sprinkle with ground cloves or ground nutmeg to taste and add sliced fresh oranges.

STUFFED ORANGES

4	large oranges
8	pitted prunes
4	teaspoons chopped walnuts
8	dried apricots, chopped
4	teaspoons golden raisins, chopped
4	(additional) dried apricots, whole, to place atop oranges

1. Slice off a small portion of the stem end of the orange. Cut triangles from the top centers.

2. Remove centers.

3. Chop the meat of the orange and combine with prunes, walnuts, raisins and chopped apricots.

4. Fill the oranges with the mixture. Top with whole dried apricot. Place oranges in a glass baking dish. Pour in enough water to cover the bottom of the dish. Bake at 300 degrees for approximately 55 minutes.

5. Put these in the oven as you begin to prepare dinner. They will be ready to eat for dessert.

Rich in the following Antioxidant Nutrients:

Vitamin A	Beta Carotene
Vitamin C	Alpha Carotene
Vitamin E	Lycopene

Plant Antioxidants:

Orange (Citrus Limonene)
Prunes
Walnuts
Apricots
Raisins

To enhance antioxidant quotient, add the following: After cooking, top with grated lemon peel and fresh ground cherries.

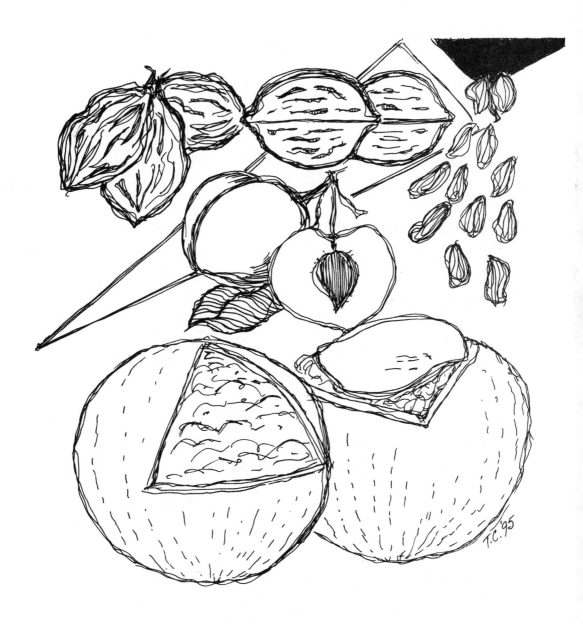

ZUCCHINI MUFFINS

1/3	cup honey
2	eggs
2	tablespoons whole wheat flour
1	teaspoon baking powder
1	teaspoon baking soda
1/2	teaspoon cinnamon
1/4	teaspoon nutmeg
1	cup grated zucchini
1/4	cup golden raisins
1/4	cup chopped walnuts

1. Beat together honey, oil and eggs.

2. Combine flour, baking powder, baking soda, cinnamon and nutmeg.

3. Combine mixtures. Add in zucchini, raisins and nuts.

4. Use paper liners in muffin tin. Spoon in batter 2/3 full. Bake in preheated 400 degree oven for 20 minutes.

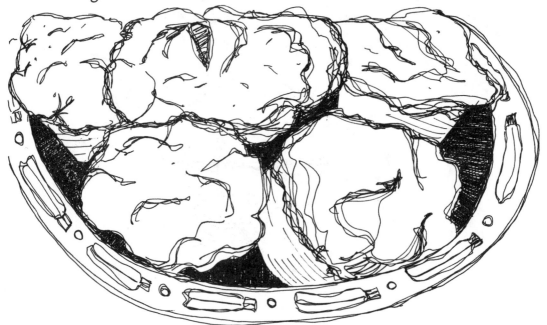

Rich in the following Antioxidant Nutrients:

Vitamin A   Beta Carotene
Vitamin C   Alpha Carotene
Vitamin E   Lycopene

Plant Antioxidants:

Walnut Oil
Whole Wheat Flour
Cinnamon
Nutmeg
Zucchini
Raisins
Walnuts

To enhance antioxidant quotient, add the following: After cooking, top with grated orange peel, ground ginger, and fresh chopped berries.

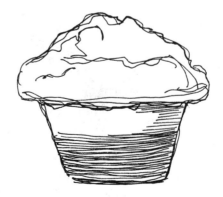

COOK'S GLOSSARY

AL DENTE: Firm to the bite

BAKE: Cooking foods by surrounding them with dry hot air.

BATONNET: Cut into sticks 1/4" x 1/4" x 3".

BLANCH: To cook item briefly in hot boiling water.

BOIL: To cook in bubbling 212 degree water.

BRAISE: To cook in a small amount of liquid. The liquid should level with the product.

BROIL: To cook with heat from above.

CHOP: To cook in irregularly sized pieces.

GRILL: To cook on an open grid over a heating source.

HERBS: The leaves of certain plants, used to flavor other foods.

JULIENNE: Cut into strips 1/8" x 1/8" x 3".

MINCE: To chop into fine pieces.

EN PAPILLOTE: (no poppy yote) Wrapped in paper for cooking. Enables foods to cook in its own juices.

POACH: Cook gently in water, or other liquid. 160 degrees.

POUND: To flatten meat with mallet or other heavy object.

PUREE: To mash, strain, process food into a smooth pulp.

REDUCE: To cook by simmering or boiling until quantity of liquid is reduced.

ROAST: To cook foods by surrounding them with hot dry air.

SAUTÉ: To cook quickly in small amount of oil.

SEAR: To brown the surface of food quickly at high temperatures.

SIMMER: To cook in water or other liquid that is bubbling gently 185 - 200 degrees.

SLICE: To cut off thin flat pieces.

SPICE: Any part of a plant, other than its leaves, used in flavoring foods.

STEAM: To cook by direct contact with steam.

SWEAT: To cook quickly in small amount of liquid that escapes from the product you are cooking.

HELPFUL HINTS

*Cutting down on fat:

  * When a recipe calls for sautéing use a non-stick, non-aluminum, stainless sauté pan.

  * When sautéing a product, get away from pouring a measured amount of oil into a pan, and use a brush. Brush the bottom, and sides of pan if needed, with oil.

  * Recommended oil per individual recipe guidelines. For coating a pan you may want to combine your oil with a flavored oil, such as sesame, peanut or walnut, depending on what you are cooking.

  * When a recipe calls for sautéing vegetables, brush the bottom of a nonstick pan with a flavorful oil. Stir in the vegetables, reduce the heat and add a couple of teaspoons of water. Cover the pan and sweat the vegetables. While doing this, stir them occasionally. This process gives you the desired result, which is to soften the vegetables. It gives a tastier result than would be achieved with steaming, and this greatly reduces the fat content produced from a sautéing process.

* About sauces.

One of the true tests of a good cooking is the ability to make a good sauce. A healthful way to make sauces is to utilize "defatted" stocks and a small amount of cornstarch to thicken them. This is done by reducing the stock down to an almost syrupy consistency, adding a little cornstarch, mixing in cold water to thicken, and then adding more broth to keep flavor and texture consistent.

Sauces can also be thickened with vegetable and fruit purees.

When using honey:

Honey is a natural sweetener. Because of its high fructose content the sweetening power of honey may be used in place of sugar. **A little math:** When baking with honey, the National Honey Board* sates that a 12 ounce jar of honey equals 1 standard measuring cup of sugar (8 ounces). So 1 ounce of sugar equals 1½ ounces of honey. A little science: You must reduce the amount of liquid (used in a standard baking recipe) by ¼ cup for each cup of honey used, due to the liquid nature of honey. When using honey in entrées and sauces, personal taste is more important than measurement! Add honey in ½ teaspoon increment. You can *always* add more, but you cannot remove what you have already blended!

* National Honey Board, Dept. CB, 421 21st Avenue, Suite 203, Longmont, CO 80501)

INDEX